Junaelo Institute Infertility Manual

Other Books by Dr. Godwin I. Meniru

A Handbook of Intrauterine Insemination. Cambridge University Press. (ISBN 0 521 58676 3).

Cambridge Guide to Infertility Management and Assisted Reproduction. Cambridge University Press. (ISBN 0 521 01071 3).

Prevention of Infertility and Complications in Women: A Comprehensive Guide to the Preservation of Female Reproductive Health. Writers Advantage Press. (Soft Cover ISBN 0 595 25722 4; Hard Cover ISBN 0 595 65282 4).

Junaelo Institute Infertility Manual

Dr. Godwin I. Meniru

M.D., M.Med.Sci., M.F.F.P., M.R.C.O.G

Medical Director
Consultant in Reproductive Medicine, Obstetrics and Gynecology
Junaelo Institute of Reproductive Medicine
Canton, OHIO

Assistant Professor of Obstetrics and Gynecology
Northeastern Ohio Universities College of Medicine
Rootstown, OHIO

iUniverse, Inc.
New York Lincoln Shanghai

Junaelo Institute Infertility Manual

iUniverse, Inc.

For information address:
iUniverse, Inc.
2021 Pine Lake Road, Suite 100
Lincoln, NE 68512
www.iuniverse.com

ISBN: 0-595-33089-4

Printed in the United States of America

Disclaimer

The author has taken care to confirm the accuracy of information that is presented in this book. However, the author and publisher make no warranty and are not responsible for any consequences that may result from the utilization of this information. Moreover, the possibility of errors, omissions, inaccuracies and inconsistencies in the information still remains for which the author and publisher cannot be held responsible. None of the parties involved in the production and marketing of this book claim to provide professional services of any sort, through the medium of this book, to individual health care practitioners, other professionals or patients. This book is not a substitute for individualized preventive and curative healthcare that is most optimally provided by physicians and their agents who are trained and certified in the relevant specialties. The opinions and information presented in this book may change in the light of future research findings, professional body and/or governmental guidelines and edicts. Drug package inserts and other authoritative up-to-date material should be consulted for current dosages, indications, side effects, complications and other concerns related to the use of specific drugs that are mentioned in this book. This book aims to educate and stimulate interest in the management of infertility. It should not be regarded as the only source of information on the matters that are discussed. The author does not seek to slight any person, group of individuals or places. Any readers who wish to apply the information in this book to their personal circumstances should use their own good judgment as well as seek expert medical opinion and guidance.

To all couples who experience difficulty in having children.

Contents

List of Tables

Acknowledgment

I wish to thank all my patients who reviewed the manuscript for this book.

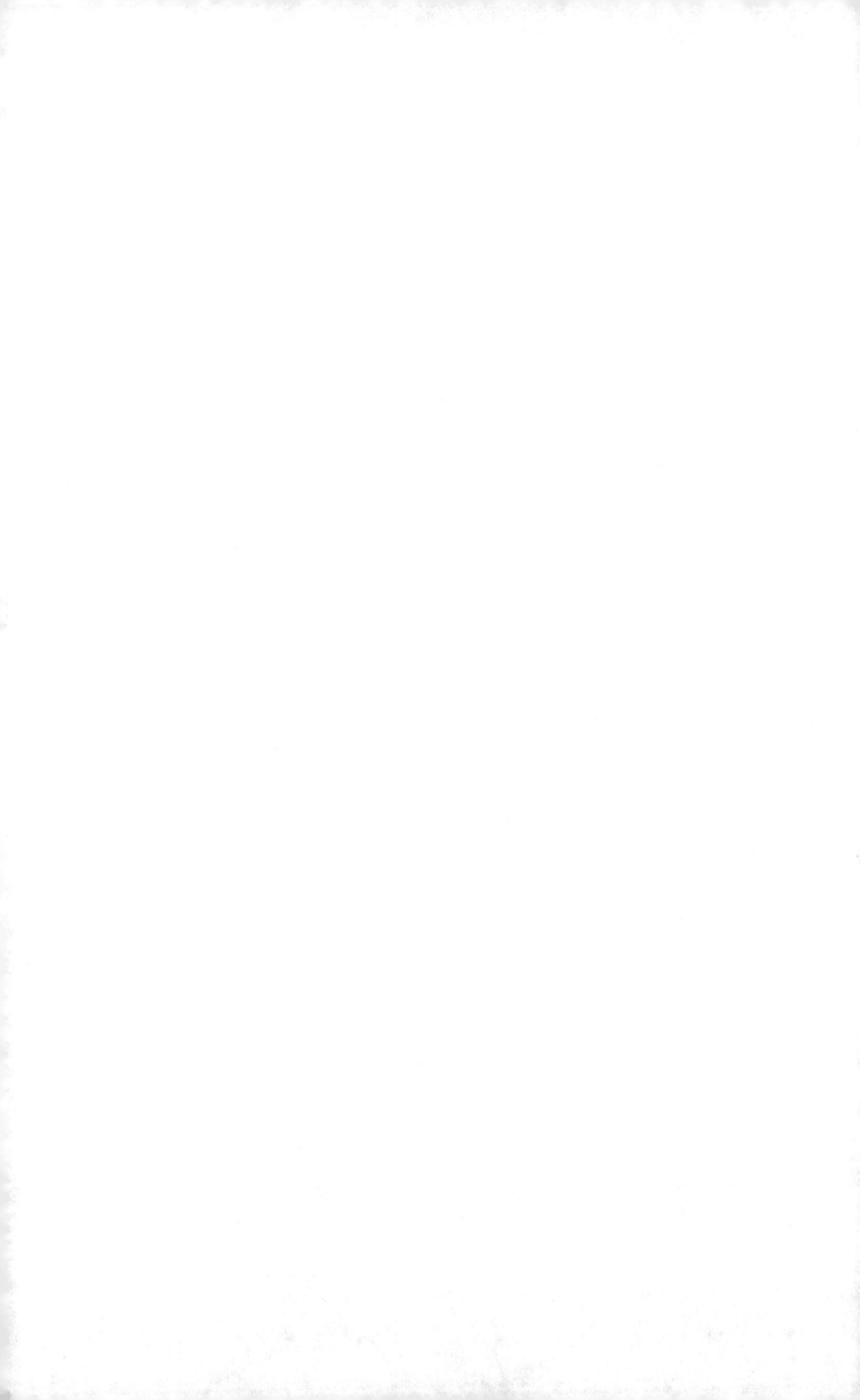

Preface

Although many couples experience delay in achieving conception mystique and ignorance still surround this common problem. One unfortunate consequence is that infertile couples are prevented from seeking timely medical evaluation and treatment. Even when they do so some patients do not know what to expect from the healthcare establishment.

This book provides simplified information on the common causes of infertility and their treatment. It is meant for anyone who is interested in gaining more knowledge of the management of infertility. This includes infertility patients themselves, their acquaintances and other motivated individuals. The book incorporates some of the initial patient teaching material that is used at Junaelo Institute of Reproductive Medicine. It also contains additional information we provide during the course of evaluation and treatment. It is meant to supplement other sources of information in the public domain including illustrated materials.

The book commences with an introduction to infertility with definitions and common concepts. This is followed by a brief description of the male and female reproductive organs; this makes it easier to understand and follow the subsequent sections. The causes of infertility are presented followed by an account of how couples are evaluated to detect or exclude the presence of infertility disorders.

The rest of the book deals with various infertility treatments that are now in common use and how they are carried out. Additional material is presented in the appendices. There is much more optimism now than there was until two decades ago regarding success following infertility treatment. Most couples can now have a reasonable expectation of achieving pregnancy. However, this may take many treatment attempts for this to happen for some couples. Furthermore, infertility treatment is invariably expensive.

It is my utmost belief that information contained in this book will ultimately benefit infertile couples. This book makes them more informed participants in the evaluation and treatment process. It also empowers them to ask for the best from their physicians. Most importantly the book tries to prepare them for the good and not so good aspects of infertility care.

Dr. Godwin I. Meniru

Junaelo Institute of Reproductive Medicine

The Junaelo Institute of Reproductive Medicine provides comprehensive infertility evaluation and treatment services. The latter services include medical and surgical treatments of infertility, induction of ovulation, intrauterine insemination, in vitro fertilization, intracytoplasmic sperm injection and gamete/embryo cryostorage. Patients who are seen at the Institute come from diverse areas; from Canton and environs, and the rest of northeastern and southeastern Ohio. The Institute also accepts patients from all over the USA and overseas.

Junaelo Institute of Reproductive Medicine provides, in addition, services in pediatric and adolescent gynecology, menopause medicine, obstetrics and gynecology, preventive women's health care and counseling.

Within the Institute is an andrology and fertility laboratory for comprehensive male fertility testing. Sperm processing for intrauterine insemination and in vitro fertilization treatment is also carried out in this laboratory together with semen freezing. Patients who are being evaluated and treated at the Institute as well as patients who are being managed by independent physicians in other facilities utilize these laboratory services.

The Institute is set to become a premier academic center majoring in preventive reproductive health care and fertility research. In collaboration with affiliated university and hospital programs the Institute participates in medical education. The publishing arm of the Institute plans to undertake production of academic texts, journals and other materials for healthcare professionals and non-medically qualified individuals.

Dr. Godwin I. Meniru is the Medical Director as well as the founder of the Institute. He is a Reproductive Medicine and Infertility Specialist. He is an

Assistant Professor of Obstetrics and Gynecology at the Northeastern Ohio Universities College of Medicine.

Contact Information

Godwin I. Meniru, M.D.
Junaelo Institute of Reproductive Medicine
4256 Fulton Drive NW Suite B, Canton, Ohio 44718
Tel: +1 330 497 9400
Fax: +1 330 497 9406
E-mail: info@JunaeloReproductiveMedicine.com
Web site: http://www.JunaeloReproductiveMedicine.com

1

Introduction to infertility

Infertility is an inability to achieve pregnancy after 1-2 years of unprotected and frequent sexual intercourse. The reason for using this time frame in defining infertility is that population studies have shown that about 80% of couples will achieve pregnancy within one year of trying. Another 10% of couples will succeed in the second year bringing the total to 90%.

This does not mean that the remaining 10% of couples will never achieve spontaneous conception. In fact another 5-7% of couples may become successful in achieving pregnancy up to the 5th year of trying for natural conception. However, using the range of 1-2 years to define infertility provides a reasonable compromise between being too conservative or aggressive in managing infertility patients.

Infertility is said to be primary if the individual has not had any pregnancy at all. Infertility is secondary if there has been a previous pregnancy, irrespective of how the pregnancy ended (e.g. miscarriage, abortion, ectopic pregnancy or stillbirth). One partner may have secondary infertility while the other partner may have primary infertility. For example, if a man previously fathered a child by another woman he is now said to have secondary infertility; if the present female partner has never been pregnant she is said to have primary infertility.

Couples who achieve pregnancies after 1-2 years of trying are said to be subfertile; their fertility is impaired to some extent but not completely. It is rare for the remaining couples from the original group (3%) to achieve conception unless some form of treatment is provided. This is because one or both members of the couple could be sterile.

Infertility therefore encompasses subfertility and sterility. Infertility is regarded as a problem of the couple. None of the partners can be said to be infertile; one or both partners may be subfertile or sterile.

There has been a marked improvement of the outcome of infertility treatment. This has now made it possible for most couples to have a reasonable expectation of becoming pregnant following treatment. There are several infertility treatments that are being used. They include medical and surgical treatments, and advanced reproductive therapies. The latter have been particularly successful in recent years.

Infertility evokes several emotions and infertile couples tend to keep quiet about their problems. There are many complex reasons for this way of behaving. Foremost is a sense of shame at being unable to reproduce naturally. In previous years and even currently, people still find it difficult discussing infertility in the open. There is still some degree of social stigma attached to infertility. Most importantly infertile couples find unkind or thoughtless utterances commonly made by other people to be deeply wounding.

Emotional support and other humane assistance will go a long way to help infertile couples cope with the reality of their experience. Provision of accurate information to the couple will assist them in making the right decision on when and where to go for medical assistance if they so wish. They also need to be well informed on what to expect from medical care. They should have an idea of how infertility is evaluated and treated, and the efficacy of various treatments. They should also understand the drawbacks and complications associated with medical intervention.

By and large the lot of infertile couples has improved in recent years. There are now several support groups who exist solely to assist infertility patients in various aspects of their care. Many professionals including physicians have made it their life's work to provide the best possible care for these individuals. However, there still remains a lot to be achieved such as making infertility care universally available and affordable.

2

The female reproductive system

Introduction

During the reproductive years, the female reproductive system is programmed to go through a regular sequence of changes in preparation for pregnancy. If pregnancy occurs, the cyclicity of these changes is interrupted; additional changes then occur in the woman's body function to maintain and support the pregnancy until delivery. A simple account of the female reproductive system is presented as an aid to understanding topics that will be discussed in later chapters.

The female sex organs

These consist of the external and internal genitalia. The external genital organs consist of the vulva. The vulva in turn is composed of the mons pubis, the clitoris, the labia minora and majora. The mons pubis is the hair bearing triangular area of skin that starts from the base of the lower abdomen and continues downwards and posteriorly where it splits into two to give rise to the labia majora.

The labia majora (singular: labium majus) are also hair bearing. They continue backwards to the perineum where they fuse. Only a relatively small distance separates the perineum from the anus. Perineum is the name given to the area of skin that lies between the vaginal opening and the anus. The labia minora (singular: labium minus) lie between the vaginal opening (introitus) and the labia majora.

The external urethral meatus lies in a triangular area of pink moist tissue called the vestibule. The base of this triangle is at the upper aspect of the vaginal introitus. The apex is bound by the labia minora as they fuse below the area of fusion of the labia majora.

The clitoris protrudes from the area that is bound above by the fusion of the labia majora and below by the fusion of the labia minora. The clitoris contains erectile tissue similar to the penis in the male.

The vagina ascends upwards and backwards from the vaginal introitus and ends at the vaginal vault. The cervix protrudes into the vagina at the vaginal vault. The upper aspect of the cervix is continuous with the uterus (womb).

Two tubular structures called the fallopian tubes arise from the upper aspects of the right and left sides of the uterus. Each tube is about 10 cm long and the outer end, which is called the infundibulum, flares out like a trumpet. The ovaries lie close to the infundibular ends of the fallopian tubes. The part of the fallopian tube that is adjacent to the infundibular end is called the ampulla. The part next to the ampulla is called the isthmus of the fallopian tube. The terminal portion of the fallopian tube (as it enters the uterine cavity) is called the interstitial part of the tube.

Ovarian cycle

Generally, every month certain changes occur in the ovaries that result in the release of an egg. All the eggs a woman will ever ovulate are present in her ovaries at the time of her birth. The eggs lay dormant in the ovaries until they commence further development that will result in either ovulation or what is called atresia. Atresia is a process of degeneration that eggs undergo if they do not make it to ovulation. This process is continuous and the ovaries lose most of their content of eggs through atresia.

Following the achievement of puberty and onset of menstruation, the woman is now capable of becoming pregnant. Eggs, which are surrounded by cells, start final developmental changes with the commencement of each menstrual period. These surrounding cells are of two major types called granulosa and theca cells. The combination of egg and surrounding cells is called a follicle. At some stage of development, fluid accumulates within the follicle and the egg comes to hang within that follicle.

Following a hormonal trigger from the pituitary gland, which is located very close to the brain, the follicle ruptures and releases the egg. This is called ovulation. The released egg, most times, is swept into the fallopian tube. Both granulosa and theca cells produce hormones such as estrogen before ovulation. Following ovulation, the follicle changes into the corpus luteum and produces estrogen as well as another hormone called progesterone.

The menstrual cycle

The uterus consists of three layers called the endometrium, myometrium and serosa. The serosa is a very thin layer that covers the outside of the uterus. The myometrium is the muscular part of the uterus and is the thickest layer. The endometrium is the innermost component of the uterus. It is also called the lining of the cavity of the uterus or endometrial lining.

The endometrium is composed of three layers too. The innermost layer is called the basal layer and is not shed during menstruation. The middle layer (spongy layer) and the uppermost layer (compact layer) are both shed during menses.

Cyclical changes occur in the endometrium every month in tandem with the ovarian changes. This is to prepare the endometrium for possible implantation of an embryo. The day of onset of menstrual bleeding is called Day 1 of the menstrual cycle. The upper layers of the endometrium are shed in the ensuing days. Menses lasts for 2-7 days usually. Following shedding of the endometrial layers and even before the bleeding stops the compact layer of the endometrium begins to regenerate the upper layers. This takes place under the influence of estrogen that is produced by the ovaries.

Further increase in the thickness and complexity of the endometrium takes place over the ensuing days. Ovulation normally occurs on Day 14 of a 28 day menstrual cycle. Following ovulation and development of the corpus luteum progesterone is produced which stimulates further developmental changes in the endometrium.

If the ovulated egg is not fertilized it disintegrates after some days. Furthermore, in the absence of fertilization, the function of the corpus luteum starts waning and production of progesterone stops. This prevents further endometrial growth; the endometrium begins to regress, and break down leading to a new menstrual period.

The hypothalamus and pituitary gland

The hypothalamus and pituitary gland are two structures that are found at the base of the brain. They perform several functions that affect various organs in the body. With respect to reproductive function, the hypothalamus produces gonadotropin releasing hormone (GnRH). This hormone stimulates the pituitary gland to secrete follicle stimulating hormone (FSH) and luteinizing hormone (LH).

The pituitary hormones have different effects on the ovary. FSH stimulates the development of ovarian follicles while LH stimulates ovulation and production of estrogen and progesterone. There is a complex interrelationship of these hormones and their actions. This is above the scope of this book but is well described in complex texts.

Conclusion

The anatomy (structure) and physiology (function) of the female reproductive system and the cyclical changes they undergo are designed to generate the female gamete (egg) and provide an environment suitable for fertilization followed by nurture of a pregnancy. Malfunction or damage to any part of this system can lead to fertility problems. Knowledge of the workings of this system makes it easier to understand how abnormalities arise and how they can be prevented and/or treated.

3

The male reproductive system

Introduction

The male reproductive organs are adapted to the function of producing sperm and transferring them to the female genital tract. In so doing, optimal conditions are created for the union of the male and female gametes. Unlike the female, production of sperm is not cyclical. Furthermore, sperm production continues well into advanced age in men, again, unlike in the female. This chapter will describe the basic structure and function of the male reproductive organs.

The male sex organs

The penis and scrotum are the visible parts of the male reproductive system. Interestingly they also house the beginning (testes) and end (penile urethra) of the male reproductive tract. The scrotum contains both testes (singular: testis) which hang outside the body cavity. This is required to keep the testes cooler than the body core temperature of 37°C. Optimal production of sperm can only take place at temperatures that are 4-7 degrees lower than the body core temperature.

Within the testes are highly coiled tiny tubes called the seminiferous tubules. Within the walls of those tubules are contained special cells called spermatogonia from which sperm are produced. The seminiferous tubules are linked through another system of tubules called the rete testis to the epididymis (plural: epididymides).

The epididymis leaves each testis as the vas deferens. The latter structure enters the body cavity through the inguinal canal that is located above the groin in the lower aspect of the abdomen. The vas deferens connects to the ejaculatory duct behind the bladder. The seminal vesicle also empties its secretions into the ejaculatory duct, which then traverses the prostate gland. The urethra originates from the bladder base and traverses the prostate gland.

The ejaculatory duct and Cowper's gland both empty into the urethra, which then enters the phallus of the penis to end at the external urethral meatus. These parts of the male reproductive system are listed in Table 3.1. It should be noted that some of the organs are paired while others are single. The accessory sex glands are the seminal vesicles, prostate and bulbo-urethral (Cowper's) glands. These produce secretions that are discharged into the male genital tract during arousal (Cowper's gland) and ejaculation (seminal vesicles and prostate).

Table 3.1. The male reproductive organs	
Components	Number
Testis	2
Excretory ducts	
Epididymis	2
Vas deferens	2
Accessory sex glands	
Seminal vesicle	2
Prostate	1
Bulbo-urethral gland	2
Ejaculatory duct	2
Urethra	1
Penis	1

Sperm production

Cells that will give rise to sperm (spermatogonia) are deposited in the testes before birth. These cells remain dormant until puberty when they begin to divide repeatedly to give rise to sperm. Four major cell stages are involved in the production of sperm—spermatogonium, spermatocyte, spermatid and spermatozoon (or sperm).

The spermatogonium divides into spermatocytes. Each spermatocyte undergoes further development to become a spermatid. The spermatid undergoes further maturation to change into a sperm. The supply of spermatogonia does not become exhausted unlike what happens to the eggs in the female. This is because not all the spermatogonia that are produced go on to become spermatocytes; some remain as spermatogonia and continue to divide into more spermatogonia and spermatocytes.

Sperm transport

At the time of production in the testes sperm do not move well; they only acquire full mobility by the time they leave the epididymis. A continuous fluid current wafts the sperm out of the seminiferous tubules until they reach the epididymides and vasa deferentia (plural of vas deferens) where they are stored.

During ejaculation, muscles found within the walls of both the epididymides and vasa deferentia contract strongly. This muscular activity propels the sperm into the ejaculatory duct and urethra. Secretions from the accessory sex glands are also discharged into the ejaculatory ducts and urethra. The mixture of sperm and the fluid derived from the accessory sex glands is called semen. This is ejected into the vagina during intravaginal ejaculation.

The hypothalamus and pituitary gland

Similar to the case in females, these organs produce hormones that influence sperm production. The hypothalamus produces gonadotropin releasing hormone. This hormone stimulates the pituitary gland to secrete follicle stimulating hormone and luteinizing hormone.

Follicle stimulating hormone stimulates the production of sperm and another hormone called inhibin from the testes. Luteinizing hormone stimulates production of testosterone, which is the "male" hormone, also from the testes.

Testosterone whilst still within the testes contributes to the stimulation of sperm production. The function of inhibin is not clear at present but it is thought to participate in "feedback" control of pituitary hormone production.

Table 3.2. Normal values of standard semen analysis

Liquefaction	Complete within 60 minutes at room temperature
Appearance	Homogenous, grey opalescent
Odor	"fresh" and characteristic
Consistency	Leaves pipette as discrete droplets
Volume	2.0 ml or more
pH	7.2 or more
Sperm concentration	20×10^6 sperm/ml or more
Total sperm count	40×10^6 sperm per ejaculate or more
Motility	50% or more sperm with forward progression (grades 'a' and 'b') or 25% or more with rapid linear progression (grade 'a') within 60 minutes of ejaculation
Morphology	30% or more spermatozoa with normal forms
Vitality	75% or more live sperm
White blood cells	Fewer than 1×10^6/ml
Immunobead test	Fewer than 50% motile sperm with beads bound
MAR test	Fewer than 50% motile sperm with adherent particles

Source:

WHO (1999)

Other aspects

- It takes about 74-78 days from the time sperm production commences in the testes to the time the sperm appears in the ejaculate.

- Semen contains cells (sperm, white blood cells and epithelial cells) and chemical constituents (water, hormones, proteins, carbohydrates, steroids, lipids) and other compounds.

- Attempts have been made to define what constitutes normal semen. The most recent proposals by the World Heath Organization are shown in Table 3.2. At present, the minimum concentration of sperm in the ejaculate that is considered as normal is 20 million sperm per milliliter.

- Semen coagulates immediately after ejaculation but liquefies within 30-60 minutes.

Conclusion

The male reproductive system is complex similar to that of the female. However, unlike the female the supply of male gametes is rarely exhausted. Furthermore, several million sperm are produced in each ejaculate while the female usually ovulates one egg in each cycle. Interestingly the causes of infertility in the female are more understood and easier to treat than in the male.

4

How conception occurs

Introduction

Conception occurs when a sperm penetrates and fuses with the egg (called fertilization) leading to the eventual production of an embryo, which burrows into the endometrium and successfully establishes contact with the mother. Fertilization of the egg is one of the key steps of reproduction. It marks the culmination of biological events some of which started or were predetermined several years previously or even before birth. It also marks the beginning of several events, which if they occur optimally may result in the delivery of a healthy baby. Any disorders that negatively influence these processes can cause infertility or pregnancy loss. This chapter describes various steps that lead to conception following sexual intercourse.

Sperm transport in the woman

Following intravaginal ejaculation, semen which is normally deposited in the upper vagina, clots but starts to liquify within 30 minutes. Right from the time of ejaculation, sperm attempt to swim out of the clot of semen. Maximal sperm escape from semen occurs after completion of liquefaction. The vaginal acidity destroys most of the sperm that are still present in the vagina after about two hours from the time of ejaculation. It is estimated that only 1% of ejaculated sperm succeed in entering the cervical canal.

In the 2-3 days preceding ovulation glands in the lining of the cervical canal produce copious amounts of clear, thin and slimy mucus. This happens because of stimulation of the glands by high estrogen levels that are usually found at this part of the menstrual cycle. The secretion is commonly called the pre-ovulatory mucus. If sexual intercourse takes place at this time, the mucus facilitates the entry of sperm into the cervical canal from where they ascend into the uterine cavity and fallopian tubes.

Some of the sperm that enter the cervical canal move to the glands in the cervical canal where they gain nourishment from the secretions. At intervals, sperm emerge from these glands and ascend the rest of the cervical canal and into the uterine cavity. This "sperm storage or buffer" phenomenon may explain why some women can become pregnant even though ovulation occurred some days after sexual intercourse. The cervix therefore acts as a sperm reservoir.

It is estimated that fertilization can occur if an egg is ovulated within 72 hours of having sexual intercourse. Fertilization is still possible if sexual intercourse occurs within 12-24 hours after ovulation. After this period, it is usually not possible for the egg to be fertilized due to aging of the egg. The cervical mucus also becomes thick and viscous due to the action of progesterone that is produced by the corpus luteum. This prevents further entry of sperm into the cervical canal from the vagina.

Fertilization

Fertilization occurs in the ampullary portion of the fallopian tube, which is adjacent to the infundibular part of the tube. Sperm has been found in the fallopian tube less than one hour after sex. Although millions of sperm are ejaculated into the vagina, only a few thousand, at the most, are found in the fallopian tube at any point in time.

Sperm that encounter the egg disperse granulosa cells that remain attached to the ovulated egg. This allows several sperm to start trying to penetrate and fertilize the egg. A single sperm eventually penetrates the outer shell of the egg (called zona pellucida) and fuses with the membrane that surrounds the egg (called the oolemma). Once this happens these barriers prevent any other sperm from penetrating and fertilizing the egg.

The first sperm to penetrate the egg fertilizes it. The fertilized egg divides into two cells within 24 hours after fertilization. These two cells (called blastomeres) are still enclosed by the zona pellucida. Once this division into blastomeres commences the fertilized egg is called an embryo. There are repeated divisions of the blastomeres as the embryo travels along the fallopian tube.

Implantation of the embryo

The embryo reaches the uterine cavity by the 5th day after ovulation. At this time, it contains several cells that were produced from the original two blastomeres and is called a morula. During the next 24 hours it changes into a blastocyst and hatches through the zona pellucida. Hatching is accomplished by the expansion of the blastocyst and secretion of chemicals that thin the zona pellucida until it cracks open.

The blastocyst also produces hormones the best known of which is human chorionic gonadotropin (HCG). The most well known action of HCG is that of preventing the demise of the corpus luteum. Human chorionic gonadotropin stimulates further production of estrogen and progesterone by the corpus luteum. The latter two hormones maintain the development of the endometrium making it possible for the embryo to implant successfully and continue development.

Following hatching, the embryo implants in the endometrium by attaching to the endometrium and literally burrowing into the endometrial layer. It then establishes contact with the mother's blood circulation through the placenta. The embryo goes through a complex series of developmental changes to become a fetus.

Conclusion

Conception occurs following the timely deposition of normal sperm in the female genital tract during the ovulatory period. Optimal egg-sperm interaction in the fallopian tube makes it possible for fertilization to take place. The embryo subsequently implants in the endometrium. At this time, the embryo has already started signaling its presence to the mother by the production of HCG and possibly other hormones. Infertility may result if any aspect of these processes becomes impaired.

5

Causes of infertility

Introduction

Although many couples may have no obvious cause for the infertility there is generally a significant incidence of infertility causing or associated factors in one or both partners. This chapter aims to present an overview of the causes of infertility. There are several outstanding books on infertility management and these should be consulted for detailed accounts of this topic. The *Cambridge Guide to Infertility Management and Assisted Reproduction* provides a comprehensive yet simple account of all aspects of infertility management.

Relative incidence of male and female infertility factors

Male factor infertility problems are found alone in 40% of cases while female factors are found in another 40%. Both male and female infertility factors are found in the remaining 20% of couples.

General overview of the causes of infertility

Several causes of infertility have been identified and are briefly described in the following sections. The man may not produce sperm at all in the testes or has very low numbers of sperm in the ejaculate. In other cases, the sperm may be of poor quality or are unable to fertilize the egg that is released every month by the woman. There may be a blockage of the male reproductive tract. This prevents sperm that are produced in the testes from being ejaculated. There can also be male or female factor problems that prevent ejaculation of semen into the vagina.

Female causes include blockage of the fallopian tubes. Some women may have problems with the production and ovulation (release) of the egg. Others may have patches of abnormal tissue, called endometriosis, in parts of their pelvis and on some of their pelvic organs. However, about 15% of couples will not have any obvious cause for their problem and are said to have "unexplained infertility".

Male factor infertility problems

- **Impotence or ejaculatory failure:** The man is unable achieve or maintain an erection of his penis. Even when an erection is achieved, he is unable to ejaculate.

- **Retrograde ejaculation:** Semen is propelled backwards into the urinary bladder instead of forwards and out of the penis during ejaculation.

- **Sexual and/or ejaculatory dysfunction:** Several disorders, including psychological factors, may render a man unable to have sexual intercourse or ejaculate.

- **Infrequent sexual intercourse:** Sex may occur so infrequently that there is no sperm present in the fallopian tube before or soon after ovulation.

- **Wrong timing of sexual intercourse:** Some couples may mistakenly have intercourse only during the non-fertile phase of the menstrual cycle.

- **Premature ejaculation:** Some men may ejaculate prematurely before inserting the penis in the vagina.

- **Extravaginal ejaculation:** This can be caused by premature ejaculation, severe hypospadias or epispadias. Due to abnormal formation, the external urethral meatus may not be located at the tip of the penis. Instead, it is located under the penile shaft (hypospadias) or above the shaft (epispadias). All these lead to the deposition of semen outside the vagina.

- **Immunologic causes:** Antibodies may be formed in the man's body and attack sperm either in the testes or after they leave the testes.

- **No demonstrable cause:** Some men may not have any obvious cause for the infertility.

- **Isolated seminal plasma abnormalities:** There may be chemical deficiencies in the fluid that surrounds the sperm. This could lead to abnormal sperm function.

- **Iatrogenic causes:** These are usually side effects of drug administration, for example, hormones, anabolic steroids, sulfasalazine, cimetidine, nitrofurantoin, niridazole, spironolactone and colchicine. Drugs that are used for treating cancer (cytotoxic drugs) especially alkylating agents (e.g. cyclophosphamide, busulphan and chlorambucil) damage testicular sperm production. Infertility can occur following prostatectomy (removal of an enlarged prostate organ), repair of inguinal hernias and hydrocelectomy. Although vasectomy is performed to prevent future pregnancies it can be regarded as a cause of infertility if in future the man decides to have more children.

- **Systemic causes:** These include diabetes mellitus, tuberculosis, high fever, general anesthesia, major surgery, burns, head injury, alcohol, other drugs of abuse, environmental toxicants, tobacco and marijuana. These either damage testicular sperm production or cause other problems such as impotence and sexual dysfunction.

- **Congenital abnormalities:** These include undescended testes and cystic fibrosis. Sperm production is either severely deficient or does not occur at all in undescended testes. Cystic fibrosis is associated with a lack of development of the vas deferens so that sperm is trapped within the testes and epididymides.

- **Acquired testicular damage:** The testes may become damaged if mumps infection affects the testes. Testicular function can also be damaged if the testis twists on its stalk and shuts off the blood supply (torsion of the testis) for more than 30 minutes.

- **Varicocele:** The veins that drain blood from the testis become dilated in this condition. This may cause sluggish drainage of blood from the testes. It is associated with impairment of testicular function.

- **Male accessory gland infection:** Infection of the accessory sex gland may impair the quality of their secretions or even block their ducts.

- **Endocrine causes:** Hypogonadotropic hypogonadism and hyperprolactinemia both lead to depressed sperm production or no production at all.

- **Unexplained poor semen parameters:** The number of sperm, their speed and pattern of movement, morphology, number of live sperm and other parameters used in judging how normal a semen sample is may become abnormal for no immediately apparent reason.

- **Obstructive azoospermia:** The vas deferens may become blocked thereby preventing sperm from being ejaculated. This can happen in men who have cystic fibrosis or are carriers of the disorder. It can also happen as a complication of certain types of surgery such as inguinal hernia repair or hydrocelectomy.

Descriptive terms for abnormal semen profiles

Azoospermia: Sperm cannot be found in a semen sample.

Aspermia: No semen was ejaculated at orgasm.

Necrozoospermia: All sperm in the semen sample are dead.

Globozoospermia: None of the sperm have acrosomal caps which are normally found on top of the sperm head and assist the sperm to penetrate the egg.

Oligozoospermia: The concentration of sperm is less than 20 million/ml of the ejaculate. This is what is normally known as "low sperm count".

Asthenozoospermia: Less than 50% of sperm in the semen sample exhibit forward motility.

Teratozoospermia: The proportion of sperm with normal shape is less than 30%.

A semen sample may at times have more than one of the last three abnormal profiles necessitating a combination of terminology. Thus oligoasthenoteratozoospermia describes a semen sample with all three abnormalities. The presence of two abnormalities will require the use of the appropriate terminology, for example, asthenoteratozoospermia.

Female factor infertility problems

Vagina

- **Coital difficulties:** Problems that prevent or limit sexual intercourse, for example, vaginismus and painful lesions of the vagina and pelvis.

Cervix

- **Mucus:** Poor mid-cycle mucus or no mucus at all.

- **Antisperm antibodies:** Antibodies directed against sperm can also be produced by the female. When present in the cervical mucus they can attack sperm and immobilize them.

- **Large number of phagocytes:** These are white blood cells. They may attack and engulf sperm that enter the cervical canal.

Uterus

- **Leiomyoma:** These are also called fibroids. They are benign tumors that are commonly found in the uterus. They usually do not cause infertility except when they distort the cavity of the uterus. Rarely they can block both tubes.

- **Endometritis:** This refers to chronic inflammation of the lining of the uterus (endometrium). This can be caused by tuberculosis. The inflamed endometrium is hostile to sperm and does not encourage implantation of the embryo.

- **Asherman's syndrome:** This occurs when damage to the endometrium leads to adherence of the walls of the uterine cavity. This can make a woman cease to have menstrual periods and/or have no free endometrial surface that is suitable for implantation of the embryo.

- **Uterine malformations:** Some types of uterine malformation can cause infertility. Others may cause menstrual abnormalities or recurrent miscarriage.

Fallopian tubes

- **Tubal blockage:** The fallopian tubes may become blocked following pelvic infection that affects the tubes.

- **Peritubal adhesions:** Scar tissue (adhesions) following infection or pelvic surgery can cover the opening of the tube preventing ovulated eggs from entering the tube. Alternatively, the adhesions may pull the tube away from the ovary so that the ovulated egg does not reach the opening of the tube.

- **Damage to tubal mucosal lining:** Damage to the inside lining of the fallopian tubes may impede the movement of sperm and/or eggs along the tube. Such injury is usually as a result of prior pelvic infection.

- **Mullerian malformations:** These refer to malformations of the fallopian tube that prevent conception. Some women may be born without one or both fallopian tubes.

- **Excised tubes due to ectopic pregnancy:** Surgical treatment of an ectopic pregnancy may involve excision of the tube together with the ectopic pregnancy.

Ovulatory disorders

- **Hypogonadotropic hypogonadism:** In this condition, there is little of no production of follicle stimulating hormone and luteinizing hormone by the pituitary gland. This means that the ovaries are not stimulated to produce eggs and hormones such as estrogen and progesterone.

- **Premature ovarian failure:** The follicles in the ovaries may become depleted before the usual age of menopause. This can happen following radiation therapy and chemotherapy for cancer. Certain infections such as mumps can also cause this problem. Certain women have antibodies that attack the follicles and damage the eggs. Some women may not have any obvious cause for their ovarian failure.

- **Polycystic ovary syndrome:** This can lead to problems with ovulation ranging from irregular ovulation to a complete lack of ovulation. It is associated with obesity, excessive hair growth on the face and body, acne, male-type baldness and several other medical problems.

- **Weight loss induced ovulatory dysfunction:** Extreme weight loss can lead to defective ovulation or a lack of ovulation. This is probably associated with the deficient amount of fat found in such women or the decrease of their body mass below a critical level. It is thought that normal ovulation occurs when a certain proportion of the body is composed of fat or when the total body mass reaches and exceeds a critical level.

- **Exercise induced ovulatory dysfunction:** Professional athletes and other women who exercise excessively also could have poor body fat stores and/or critically low body mass leading to ovulatory problems.

- **Hyperprolactinemia:** This refers to the presence of high levels of prolactin in the blood stream. Prolactin is a hormone that is produced in the pituitary gland. Hyperprolactinemia can be due to pregnancy, breast feeding, brain tumors or medications. The high prolactin level interferes with ovulation. At times, there is no obvious cause for the high prolactin levels. There are several other causes of hyperprolactinemia that are not mentioned here.

Other problems

- **Endometriosis:** This is a condition in which tissue that appears similar to the endometrium is found in sites other than the endometrial layer of the uterus. Such sites include the pelvis or other parts of the body. It may be mild/minimal, moderate or severe. It is not certain if mild/minimal endometriosis causes infertility.

- **No detectable problem:** Similar to the male, there are females in whom no obvious cause for the infertility is found even after extensive investigation.

Conclusion

Students of reproductive biology often marvel not at why infertility occurs but why people get pregnant in the first place. This is because human reproduction is a very delicate process. It involves apparent chance events such as viable sperm being present in the fallopian tubes when the ovulated egg reaches there. It is therefore no surprise that several factors can cause infertility. However, knowledge of the causes of infertility helps physicians plan an adequate evaluation of infertile couples. It also helps patients understand and follow their management.

6

Evaluation of infertility

Introduction

A couple can seek medical opinion and possible treatment whenever they become sufficiently anxious about their continued inability to achieve pregnancy. Some may do so after one or two years of trying while others may wait for much longer. However, there is nothing wrong with any couple consulting a physician earlier than this; it is better to be early rather than late.

It is not necessary for the physician to treat everyone who consults him. His first emphasis is to find out if there is a cause for the infertility. He will ask the couple several questions, examine them, carry out some laboratory tests and other investigations (see Appendices I-V).

If a problem is detected it then means that the couple have benefited by presenting early to the doctor. If no cause is found, some couples may become less anxious and continue trying to get pregnant by natural means, provided the woman's age is not of concern. Some couples may take longer than others to achieve natural conception.

Basic infertility investigations

Investigations (Table 6.1) can be completed within 1-2 months. It is advisable to carry out semen analysis first since the result may influence the pattern of the woman's investigations. For example, a severely abnormal semen analysis result may mean that the woman does not need to have a test to check for whether her fallopian tubes are open, such as hysterosalpingography or the laparoscopy and dye test operation. This is because the couple invariably will require advanced reproductive therapy, such as in vitro fertilization and intracytoplasmic sperm injection, that does not require the presence of patent fallopian tubes. In such instances, checking for tubal patency will be of no utility. Tests of tubal patency are described in detail in Appendices II-IV.

However, some couples may decide to use donor sperm for artificial insemination if the man's semen profile is severely abnormal or the man has no sperm in his ejaculate (azoospermia). In such cases, tubal patency has to be confirmed before proceeding with the treatment.

Semen analysis is one of the easiest and least expensive tests to perform for infertile couples. It is also not invasive. The semen sample is produced by masturbation after abstaining from ejaculation for 2-5 days (see Appendix V).

The woman should still have investigations such as hormone assay irrespective of the man's semen analysis result, provided the couple wish to have treatment. Hormone assay means the measurement of the level (or concentration) of hormones in blood. Hormone assay is performed on Day 2, 3, 4, or 5 of the menstrual cycle. Hormones that are assayed include follicle stimulating hormone (FSH), luteinizing hormone (LH), prolactin, estrogen and thyroid stimulating hormone.

Hormone assay can also be required for the man if the semen analysis result is abnormal. Hormones that are commonly assayed in men include FSH, LH, testosterone and prolactin.

Hysteroscopy involves the use of a small "telescope-like" device to look inside the uterine cavity. It is performed under general or local anesthesia. During the procedure, a careful search of the uterine cavity is carried out looking for problems such as protruding fibroids or polyps.

Pelvic ultrasonography and saline infusion sonography (SIS) are used to evaluate the size of the uterus and contour of the uterine cavity respectively. Again, this is mainly for visualizing fibroids but endometrial polyps can be seen on occasions. Polyps are structures that hang in the uterine cavity suspended from their attachment to the endometrium.

During SIS, fluid is slowly injected into the uterine cavity using a small polythene or rubber tube (cannula) that is passed through the cervical canal. An ultrasound scan of the uterus is performed simultaneously using a probe that is inserted into the vagina. The fluid distends the uterine cavity making it easier to see polyps or any other structure that distorts the shape of the uterine cavity.

The post-coital test is used to check for the survival of sperm in the cervical mucus. It is performed at the middle of the menstrual cycle (mid-cycle), at the time of production of the pre-ovulatory mucus. The couple is asked to have sexual intercourse on the night before the test. The woman should not douche afterwards. She reports to the physician on the following morning. A sample of mucus is gently aspirated from her cervical canal using a small syringe that is attached to a plastic tube. This mucus is spread on a glass slide and examined under the microscope for the presence of live motile sperm.

Table 6.1. Basic infertility investigations
Semen analysis
Hormone assay of the male partner if required
Hormone assay of the female partner
Tests of tubal patency
• Hysterosalpingography (HSG)
• Hysterosalpingocontrast sonography (HyCoSy)
• Laparoscopy and dye test
Testing for the occurrence of ovulation (see Table 6.2)
Hysteroscopy if required
Pelvic ultrasound scan
Saline infusion sonography
Post-coital test

Detection of ovulation

There is no direct method of documenting ovulation. Indirect methods that are commonly used are shown in Table 6.2. When the clinical history is obtained an idea is gained as to whether the woman ovulates regularly. A woman who has regular menstrual periods every month is likely to be ovulating regularly.

The body temperature can be measured first thing in the morning before getting out of bed. Ovulation is predicted by a small drop in the body temperature that is followed by a rise of half a degree (Centigrade). This rise is maintained for about 10 days before dropping back to normal levels. This is called basal body temperature measurement. This method may not reliably detect the occurrence of ovulation in every patient. However, it may be useful in some women especially when combined with other monitoring techniques.

Cervical mucus becomes profuse, thin, clear, slippery, and can stretch into a thread at mid-cycle just before ovulation. Following ovulation the mucus becomes thick, whitish and scanty due to the action of progesterone.

A strip of the endometrium can be obtained from the uterus four days before the predicted date of the next menstrual period. This is examined under the microscope. If ovulation had occurred in that menstrual cycle, characteristic microscopic "secretory" changes will be seen in the endometrial tissue.

The development of ovarian follicles and increase in thickness of the endometrium can both be monitored using ultrasound scanning. Following ovulation the follicle will be seen to have disappeared, to be replaced by the corpus luteum. The endometrium will also show signs of the action of progesterone which is now being produced by the corpus luteum.

Measuring the progesterone level on Day 21 of the cycle is the most convenient way of documenting ovulation. The progesterone level usually becomes elevated following ovulation.

The woman can test her urine each day using a test kit that she is provided with. This kit will detect the surge of luteinizing hormone production that precedes ovulation by about 36-40 hours.

The importance of female age

It is important for the age of the woman to be kept in mind when making decisions regarding infertility assessment and treatment. This is because the natural decline in the fertility of females accelerates from about 35 years onwards. By age 42 years and above it will be much more difficult for the woman to become pregnant naturally. It will also be difficult for any assisted conception treatment using her eggs to succeed after this age. A pragmatic approach should be adopted especially for females aged 35 and above; rapid assessment is required and the best available treatment offered immediately.

Table 6.2. Techniques for determining the occurrence of ovulation

Monitoring changes in basal body temperature during the menstrual cycle

Detecting cervical mucus changes at mid-cycle

Endometrial biopsy just before the next menstrual period

Ultrasonography of the ovaries and endometrium

Day 21 progesterone assay to confirm that ovulation occurred on Day 14

Luteinizing hormone surge detection. (Ovulation usually follows the surge)

Female fertility

The female is born with all the eggs she will ever ovulate already present in her ovaries. However, the number of eggs begins to decrease, without being ovulated, from her fifth month in the womb. The depletion of eggs occurs through a process that is known as atresia. By the time she is 25 years old she only has about 60,000 eggs remaining in her ovaries. By 40 years 8,000 eggs remain.

As more eggs degenerate in the ovary and the woman becomes older, her fertility drops. This is because the eggs remaining in the ovaries are older and do not respond well to the stimulus provided by FSH and LH. Both of these hormones are produced by the pituitary gland. In an attempt to improve on the poor ovarian response, the pituitary produces more FSH and LH. This does not have the desired effect and fewer eggs are still ovulated.

There comes a time when ovarian response is so poor that no more eggs are ovulated. Normally this should occur when the woman is about 50 years old. The menstrual periods stop and the woman is said to be menopausal. Ovarian failure is normal in this context because it occurs at the expected age. If however, ovarian failure occurs before the age of 40 years it is said to be premature.

Conclusion

Evaluation of infertile couples can detect obvious infertility factors such as blocked tubes, problems with ovulation, endometriosis and abnormal semen parameters. It can also identify or exclude many other factors when the patient's medical history is obtained and during physical examination. Infertility problems that are detected can then be treated if possible. Couples in whom no infertility factor is apparent can either be managed expectantly or offered advanced reproductive therapy. These treatments will be discussed in subsequent chapters.

7

An overview of infertility treatments

Introduction

Irrespective of whether a cause is found for the state of infertility or not, there comes a time when the couple may decide to seek treatment. The timing depends on each couple but is usually related to their response to the following questions:

- How long have they been trying?

- How long are they prepared to continue trying?

- What is the woman's age?

- When can they afford the cost (financial, emotional, time off work) of treatment?

Infertility treatment can be medical, surgical or by advanced reproductive therapy. Medical and surgical treatment can be carried out for a select few infertility problems. Advanced reproductive therapy can be used for the remaining couples who often have a wide range of infertility problems; it can also be used when no obvious cause for the infertility is found.

Medical treatment of infertility

Medication can be given to some couples to improve the sperm quality, make the woman ovulate or treat some other causes of infertility such as endometriosis. However, few men with sperm quality problems will show any improvement with drug treatment.

Surgical treatment of infertility

Poor sperm quality in some men with varicose veins of the testes (varicocele) may improve after the veins are tied off at operation. Women with blocked fallopian tubes may become pregnant when the tubes are opened surgically. Destroying the endometriotic deposits with laser or cautery may lead to natural conception in some women. Again, only a few problems can be treated successfully with surgery.

Advanced reproductive therapy (assisted conception treatment)

This name is given to any treatment that seeks to bring the eggs and sperm close together. This is in an attempt to improve the chances of fertilization and the occurrence of pregnancy. There are several such treatments. Some are more sophisticated, invasive and expensive than others. The particular treatment to apply to a couple depends on the specific features of their problem. Commonly used assisted conception treatments are shown in Table 7.1.

Ovulation induction

The woman is given drugs such as clomiphene citrate tablets or gonadotropin injections to make her produce one egg. The couple then have sexual intercourse around the predicted time of ovulation. This treatment is usually given to females who have ovulatory problems that are amenable to treatment e.g. polycystic ovary syndrome and hypogonadotropic hypogonadism.

Table 7.1. Advanced reproductive therapies

Induction of ovulation

Artificial insemination

- Intrauterine insemination (IUI)

- Intravaginal insemination

- Peri-cervical insemination

- Intracervical insemination

- Intratubal insemination

- Direct intraperitoneal insemination

- Direct intrafollicular insemination

In vitro fertilization (IVF)

Intracytoplasmic sperm injection (ICSI)

Embryo freezing and frozen embryo replacement

Gamete intrafallopian transfer (GIFT)

Zygote intrafallopian transfer (ZIFT)

Surgical sperm retrieval

Intrauterine insemination (IUI)

The woman is administered drugs to make her produce and ovulate 2-4 eggs. The partner provides a sample of his semen. This is prepared in the laboratory to select out the motile normal shaped sperm. The suspension of prepared sperm is gently injected into the woman's womb. The expectation here is that sperm will fertilize some of the ovulated eggs inside the woman's fallopian tubes. Other types of artificial insemination are listed in Table 7.1. Further information on IUI is provided in Chapter 8 as well as in Appendices VI and VII.

In vitro fertilization (IVF) treatment

The woman is administered drugs to make her produce many eggs (up to 10-15 eggs at times). A special needle is used to aspirate the eggs from her ovaries about an hour before the eggs are due to be ovulated. These eggs are put into special dishes containing culture medium and placed inside incubators.

The man provides a semen sample, which is washed with gamete culture medium to select out only the live normal motile sperm. A measured volume of the washed sperm suspension is mixed with the eggs. Fertilized eggs are removed the following day and put into a fresh culture dish. After 1-4 more days in the incubator 1-3 embryos are gently placed in the woman's womb. Some of the remaining embryos may be frozen for possible use in future if their quality is assessed to be good. A detailed account of IVF treatment is given in Chapter 9 and Appendices X-XIII.

Intracytoplasmic sperm injection (ICSI)

This treatment is used in addition to IVF for men who have very poor quality sperm. A live sperm is picked up with a tiny needle and injected into each egg. Some of these eggs then go on to fertilize. The rest of the treatment is similar to IVF. Further details on ICSI treatment are provided in Chapter 10.

Frozen embryo replacement

Frozen human embryos have now being used for treating infertile couples for many years. They have resulted in the birth of several thousand healthy babies. Excess embryos resulting from IVF treatment or ICSI can be frozen after 1-5 days in culture. Following thawing these embryos are replaced in the uterus at the correct time in relation to ovulation and the thickness of the lining of the uterus (endometrium). Additional information on frozen embryo replacement is provided in Chapter 11 and Appendix XVII.

Gamete or zygote intrafallopian transfer

These procedures are not commonly performed now. Eggs are collected from the woman. Two to three eggs are mixed with a suspension of washed sperm and put back in the woman's fallopian tubes. The expectation here is that the eggs will become fertilized inside the tubes just as happens naturally. This technique is called gamete intrafallopian transfer (GIFT).

Alternatively, IVF (or ICSI) is carried out initially. Two to three fertilized eggs are then replaced in the fallopian tubes the next day. These embryos are carried down the fallopian tubes by the movement of the tubes and eventually reach the uterine cavity where they implant. This technique is called zygote intrafallopian transfer (ZIFT).

Surgical sperm retrieval

As already noted some men may have a block somewhere along their reproductive tract. This prevents sperm that have already been produced in the testes from appearing in the ejaculate. Sperm can be aspirated from the testis or epididymis of such men and used for ICSI. Surgical sperm retrieval methods are listed in Table 7.2.

Table 7.2. Surgical sperm retrieval methods and some acronyms.

Technique	Acronym
Percutaneous epididymal sperm aspiration	PESA
Microepididymal sperm aspiration	MESA
Testicular sperm aspiration	TESA
Testicular sperm extraction	TESE
Vas deferens sperm aspiration	-
Rete testis aspiration	-
Spermatocele aspiration	-
Sperm reservoir	-

Percutaneous epididymal sperm aspiration (PESA) is the least invasive of these procedures. It successfully retrieves sperm from the epididymis of men with obstructive azoospermia in 80-100% of cases. PESA should be the procedure of first choice due to its simplicity.

PESA is performed by inserting a needle through the skin of the scrotum and into the epididymis followed by aspiration with a syringe. The recovered sperm are processed in the laboratory and used for treating the infertile couple immediately and/or frozen for future use. PESA is performed under anesthesia. The patient should not feel any pain during the procedure and goes home on that same day.

If PESA is not successful, any of the other techniques can be tried. In testicular sperm aspiration (TESA) a needle is pushed into the testis and used in aspirating a small amount of testicular tissue. In testicular sperm extraction (TESE) an incision is made into the testis to allow the removal of a larger amount of testicular tissue. Testicular tissue is processed in the laboratory to extract the sperm.

Microepididymal sperm aspiration (MESA) involves the use of an operating microscope to identify the tiny epididymal tubules, which are opened, and their contents aspirated. A scrotal incision is required.

Success rates of advanced reproductive therapies

The chance of pregnancy occurring after any one of these treatments depends on the particular treatment method used and other factors such as the age of the woman and the cause of the infertility. The pregnancy rate may range from 10-50% or more in each cycle of treatment. If the couple have repeated cycles of assisted conception treatment, their cumulative chance of achieving a pregnancy also increases. Some may achieve a cumulative pregnancy rate of 40-90% or more in one year of 3-4 treatment cycles.

Counseling and information

Infertile couples need to be highly informed on fertility matters. They should be encouraged to read books and other sources of information. Counseling and psychological support should be provided to them, as this is a very difficult phase in their life.

Infertility evokes profound psychological reactions in affected couples and alters their perception of life. One of the notable features is that of feeling intensely alone. Assisted conception treatments are complex and stressful. There is need for support, and counseling facilities are provided.

Couples are ideally seen by the counselor prior to commencing treatment, during the treatment and afterwards especially if the treatment fails. The role of counseling in assisted conception treatments cannot be overemphasized.

Conclusion

Of the existing therapies for infertility, advanced reproductive therapy (ART) currently offers the most pragmatic and cost effective option. Traditional medical and surgical treatments are of limited value. The relatively high cost of assisted conception treatments prevents a significant proportion of couples from seeking such treatments especially as insurance coverage for ART is not universal.

8

Intrauterine insemination

Introduction

Intrauterine insemination (IUI) is an assisted conception treatment method that can be used to treat infertility in certain groups of patients. It involves the deposition of a washed sample of sperm in the uterine cavity around the predicted time of ovulation. Usually the woman's ovaries are stimulated to produce 2-4 eggs.

These manipulations have certain advantages over the natural situation. Firstly, many more sperm are spared from destruction in the vagina and they are directly placed in the uterus. Secondly, the distance the sperm has to travel to reach the site of fertilization in the fallopian tube is greatly shortened. Thirdly, more eggs are available in the fallopian tubes and this increases the chances of, at least one of them, being fertilized. Finally, the presence of more than one embryo likewise improves the chances of one of them implanting in the uterus.

Intrauterine insemination is one of the simpler and less expensive assisted conception treatment methods. It is also effective. However, it cannot be used for every couple with infertility.

Couples who are not suitable candidates for IUI

Not every couple with infertility is a suitable candidate for IUI. For example, those with blocked fallopian tubes cannot become pregnant through IUI since the procedure requires normal functioning fallopian tubes. Women who have reached their menopause (either naturally or prematurely) will not respond to ovarian stimulation.

Men with severe sperm abnormalities and couples with complex infertility problems should have treatment with other assisted conception methods such as in vitro fertilization (IVF).

Contraindications to treatment with IUI include infection of the woman's genital tract (cervix, uterus, fallopian tubes) or pelvis. Unexplained abnormal bleeding and the presence of large tumors in the pelvis are other reasons for not performing IUI. These conditions should first be treated after which IVF rather than IUI should be performed.

Couples who can have IUI

Although not an exhaustive list, couples with any of the following fertility problems or diagnoses may be suitable for IUI:

- Impotence or ejaculatory problems.

- Mildly abnormal sperm samples.

- Antisperm antibodies.

- Infrequent sexual intercourse.

- Cervical mucus abnormalities.

- Certain types of ovulatory problems.

- Endometriosis.

- Unexplained infertility.

- Other problems and indications.

Steps in the treatment

- Stimulation of the ovaries using clomiphene citrate tablets and/or gonadotropin injections.

- Ultrasound scanning to monitor the woman's response to ovarian stimulation.

- Prediction of the occurrence of ovulation by daily testing of urine samples starting from Day 9 or 10.

- Human chorionic gonadotropin (HCG) injection is used to trigger ovulation or support the body's own attempt to trigger ovulation.

- The man's sperm are washed in the laboratory and placed in the woman's uterus on 1-2 consecutive days around the time of ovulation.

- See Appendices VI and VII for further details.

Success rates

About 10-15% of couples will become pregnant in each cycle of treatment. Most couples who get pregnant using IUI usually do so within the first four cycles of treatment. These four cycles can often be completed within a period of 8-12 months. It is not advisable to continue treatment with IUI after this number of attempts. Instead, the patient should consider having IVF treatment.

Complications

Complications are not common following treatment with IUI. Infection may occur in 0.2% of couples. Allergic reaction to constituents of the sperm washing fluid can occur but this is rare. The incidence of multiple pregnancy is increased (11-30% of pregnancies) because the ovaries are stimulated to produce more than one egg. The ovaries may become overstimulated in about 1% of cases leading to ill health that may last for two weeks or more. This is called ovarian hyperstimulation syndrome. Some studies have suggested that the risk of developing ovarian cancer is higher in women who have ovarian stimulation. However, there is still no definite proof that this happens.

Conclusion

Intrauterine insemination is a more affordable advanced reproductive therapy that is suitable for patients with certain types of infertility problems. However, treatment attempts should not exceed four as success after this becomes more difficult to predict.

It is important that the couple understands all aspects of IUI before making a decision to have the treatment. Additional information can be found in *A Handbook of Intrauterine Insemination*, Cambridge University Press, Cambridge.

9

In vitro fertilization

Introduction

In vitro fertilization (IVF) treatment is one of the assisted conception treatments for infertility. Due to its complexity, it is important that couples are made aware of all aspects of the treatment. This improves their compliance since they know exactly what to expect and when.

Most importantly, they are fully informed on issues such as the number of embryos to replace, success rate of the treatment, complications and side effects that are possible.

This account has been written with the objective of imparting as much factual information as possible to the couple in a format that is easy to understand. It is hoped that it will supplement other sources of information available to couples who are preparing to have IVF treatment.

Manipulation of menstrual cycles

In vitro fertilization treatment is carried out at set times during the year in many centers. However, not every woman will be at the required phase of the menstrual cycle at these times. Therefore, there may be a need to readjust the menstrual cycles of such women so that all patients start having their menstrual periods at the required time.

The manipulation of menstrual cycles involves the use of medications such as progesterone, medroxyprogesterone acetate (Provera), or oral contraceptive tablets. These can either be used to postpone the onset of the next menstrual period or bring it forward. Some patients may not need these medications since they will already be at the right phase of the menstrual period.

In other centers, IVF treatment is carried out virtually every day. In such places it is not necessary to synchronize the menstrual cycles of the patients. Each patient commences IVF treatment without reference to the menstrual cycles of other women in the program.

Gonadotropin releasing hormone agonists

Gonadotropin releasing hormone agonists (GnRHa) are drugs that are used in preventing the pituitary gland from interfering with the function of the ovaries during ovarian stimulation. Normally, the pituitary gland, which is located in the lower part of the brain, controls how the ovaries function.

The pituitary gland does this by producing two hormones called follicle stimulating hormone (FSH) and luteinizing hormone (LH). The level of these hormones is controlled by the pituitary gland such that it is just adequate for the growth and ovulation of one egg. During IVF treatment, the ovaries are stimulated with larger doses of FSH and LH, which are administered as daily injections. This is aimed at the production of 10-20 eggs.

The pituitary gland also stimulates the release of the mature egg by suddenly increasing the production of LH. This is called the 'LH surge' and it occurs about 36-40 hours before ovulation. During IVF treatment, the eggs have to be aspirated from the ovaries before ovulation occurs. This is another reason why it is important to block the pituitary from initiating an LH surge before the eggs are ready for collection.

There are several GnRHa preparations that can be used to suppress pituitary function. They may be administered as injections (e.g. Lupron, Lupron Depot and Zoladex). They can also be administered as intranasal sprays such as Nafarelin (Synarel).

Nafarelin is sprayed into one nostril in the morning and in the other nostril in the evening i.e. 12 hours apart. Zoladex and Lupron Depot only need to be administered once (as a depot injection). Zoladex injection is given into the fat layer of the anterior abdominal wall below the umbilicus. One dose of this injection lasts for 28 days. Lupron Depot lasts for 30 days. However, the other preparation of the same compound, Lupron, is administered as a daily intramuscular injection.

The administration of GnRHa is commenced from either Day 2 or Day 21 of the menstrual cycle. The patient will be told exactly when to start. It will take an average of 10-14 days for the pituitary gland to be sufficiently suppressed. Maintenance of pituitary suppression is generally required for an additional two weeks.

In some cases GnRHa may be given for longer than 10-14 days before starting gonadotropin injections. This happens in some patients in whom it is difficult to program the menstrual cycle with progesterone, Provera, oral contraceptive tablets or similar medications. The GnRHa is continued for 21 days, 28 days or any number of days required for the woman reach the stage when gonadotropin injections can be started. Those who are currently on GnRHa treatment for endometriosis (GnRHa is usually administered for 3-6 months) can even start IVF treatment without waiting for regular menstrual periods to return.

Gonadotropin releasing hormone antagonists

These antagonists to pituitary production and release of FSH and LH are relatively new in clinical practice. Their administration leads to immediate suppression of the pituitary gland thereby preventing premature ovulation. There are two preparations of these compounds that are currently in use: Cetrorelix and Ganirelix. They are administered as daily injections starting after about 6-7 days of administering FSH injections.

Gonadotropin injections

About 10-14 days after commencing GnRHa treatment, daily injections of gonadotropins are commenced. There are many gonadotropin preparations. Some contain mainly FSH while others contain a mixture of LH and FSH. Currently available preparations include Fertinex, Follistim, Gonal-F, Humegon, Pergonal and Repronex.

The dose of gonadotropin that is administered to any particular patient depends on a number of factors. These include age, build, dose used in previous treatment cycles, whether the ovaries are polycystic, and if she had ovarian hyperstimulation syndrome in a previous treatment cycle.

The dose may have to be increased or decreased depending on the woman's response to the administered drugs. Some women may receive 150 international units (IU) a day while others will receive 225 IU. Some older women may require up to 450 IU daily to stimulate development of the follicles in the ovaries. A follicle is a fluid filled bag within which the egg develops in the ovary. Gonadotropin injections are continued until the follicles in the ovaries have reached the right size. The injections are usually given for 12-21 days.

Human chorionic gonadotropin injection

Since the natural LH surge is abolished by the use of GnRHa or antagonists, alternative ovulation triggers are required. The LH surge commences final maturation of the egg and this is an important step in the development of eggs in the ovaries.

Human chorionic gonadotropin (HCG) is a hormone that shares some similarities with LH; it can induce similar maturation in developing eggs. An injection of 10,000 IU of HCG is administered when the developing follicles have reached the required size. The eggs are aspirated from the ovaries about 34-36 hours after the hCG injection. The brand names of available hCG preparations are Novarel, Ovidrel and Profasi. The administration of GnRHa is stopped once HCG is injected.

Ultrasound scans

Ultrasound scanning is the main method of monitoring the woman's response to ovarian stimulation. Most of the scanning will be carried out transvaginally because that gives the best image of the pelvic organs. The ultrasound probe is covered with one or two disposable rubber sheaths before being gently introduced into the vagina and used in scanning the pelvis.

An initial ultrasound scan is carried out 10-14 days after commencing GnRHa treatment. This is to confirm that there are no cysts or any other abnormalities of the ovaries. The lining of the inside of the womb is also examined to make sure it is thin and looks normal.

The next ultrasound scan will be scheduled to take place after 6-8 days of gonadotropin injections. Subsequently, scans are carried out daily or every other day depending on the response. On each occasion the ovaries and uterus are examined. The number of developing follicles in each ovary is checked and their size measured.

Hormone assays

The concentration of certain hormones for example, estrogen and LH, may be measured through blood tests that are carried out 10-14 days after commencing GnRHa treatment. This is to make sure that adequate control has been achieved over pituitary function. Subsequent hormone assays measure mainly estrogen which is produced by the ovaries.

The estrogen level can give an indication of how well the ovaries are responding to the stimulation. It will also indicate whether the woman is over-responding to the gonadotropin injections. These hormone assays may not be carried out on every patient as ultrasound scanning gives information that is more useful.

Egg retrieval

The patient reports to the fertility center on the morning of the procedure. She should be fasting for at least five hours; she is usually advised not to have food or drink from the preceding midnight. She is prepared in the receiving room of the Center and taken to the IVF procedure room.

Intravenous injections of strong analgesics and sedatives are administered. These will make the patient drowsy or sleep off during the procedure. A transvaginal ultrasound scan is carried out and eggs are aspirated from follicles in both ovaries. This is achieved through the use of a hollow needle which pierces the vaginal wall and punctures the follicles.

The eggs are placed in special plastic dishes containing a solution that is rich in nutrients (called culture medium). These dishes are maintained in an incubator at a temperature that is similar to that of the body (i.e. 37 degrees centigrade).

Eggs can also be aspirated from the ovaries using a laparoscope. This is inserted into the abdomen through an incision that is made just below the umbilicus. However, the vaginal route of egg collection is preferred nowadays. Following completion of the egg recovery procedure an antibiotic is administered to help prevent pelvic infection.

Transvaginal egg collection is a relatively safe procedure. The patient should not feel pain and she wakes up soon afterwards. The procedure takes an average of 30 minutes. After a short while in the IVF center, the patient is usually discharged home on that same day.

Before discharge, the findings at operation are discussed with the couple and they are informed of the number of eggs that were collected. It is very important that the patient confirms her current phone numbers so that she can be contacted whenever required during the next five days. The patient should not drive a vehicle for 24 hours after the procedure. She must be driven home by her partner or an acquaintance.

Production of a semen sample

The patient's partner is required to produce a semen sample that will be used to fertilize the eggs. The sample is produced at the same time as the egg retrieval is being carried out. This arrangement makes it possible for the man to be with his partner until she goes in for the egg retrieval; he then goes and produces the sample and is back before she comes out of the procedure room.

Alternatively, he can produce the sample before the partner goes in for the egg collection especially if there are other patients scheduled to have the procedure before her. The semen sample is produced by masturbation after 2-3 days of abstinence from ejaculation. A specific instruction for the man therefore is to ejaculate (through sexual intercourse or masturbation) 3 days before the expected date of egg collection.

The quality of the semen sample may become poor if the period of abstinence is more than 7-10 days. The ejaculate is collected into well-labeled sterile plastic containers that are non-toxic to sperm. It is recommended that the man washes his hands and genitals with soap, rinses them several times with clean water and dries with a clean towel. No lubricant such as petroleum jelly is allowed during masturbation since most of these lubricants have been shown to be toxic to sperm.

Difficulty with producing semen samples

It is preferable to produce this sample within the laboratory premises. However, some men may find it difficult to masturbate on demand in strange environments. Such people can produce the sample at home and bring it in immediately. The sample should reach the laboratory within 30-60 minutes of production.

Care should be taken to keep the semen sample warm. However, it should not rest on hot surfaces such as domestic heaters since the sperm will die immediately. The container can be carried in a shirt pocket close to the skin in cold climates. In warm climates, hot areas are avoided. Again, the sample is carried on the person and taken to the laboratory as soon as possible.

Rooms are specially set aside in fertility centres or laboratories for production of semen samples by masturbation. Such rooms are ideally located in a quiet part of the unit. Suitable magazines and video recordings are normally provided in these rooms for those who require them.

Some men may find it impossible to masturbate because of psychological reasons. Such men are provided with special condoms to use for sexual intercourse at home. These are not the usual condoms that are available in shops and supermarkets that contain chemicals that kill sperm; rather, they are made of silastic rubber material that has been found not to be toxic to sperm. Following ejaculation, the condom is carefully removed from the penis and the semen emptied into the sterile jar that is provided.

There are still other men who cannot produce a semen sample, with any of these methods, on demand. They are provided with containers to keep at home. They are asked to masturbate into one of the containers on any day they choose and bring in the sample. The semen sample is analyzed and frozen for use during future IVF treatment cycles.

Obviously, such patients have to be identified before hand for this strategy to be usefully applied for future IVF treatments. If this problem is only detected on the day of egg collection one of the options would be to cancel the IVF treatment at that stage. Alternatively, sperm can be aspirated with needles from the man's epididymis and/or testes.

Whole versus split ejaculates

Semen can be collected as a whole or split ejaculate. The man will be told which type will be required. In the first type, the whole of the ejaculate is collected into one container and analyzed as such. In the second type, the man is given two containers that are held together with adhesive tape.

One of the containers is labeled as '1' while the other is labeled '2'. The man is instructed to commence ejaculation into 'Pot 1' and, after the first two spurts, to move on to 'Pot 2' where he is to finish the ejaculation. The reason for using this method of collection is that most of the ejaculated sperm can be found in the first one or two spurts while the remaining part of the ejaculate consists mainly of fluid from the various accessory sex glands.

The samples in the two pots are analyzed separately and the results combined. Split ejaculate is required by some fertility units while other units use whole ejaculates for analysis and assisted conception treatments.

The semen sample is analyzed and then prepared for use in IVF. Different methods of sperm preparation are in use. All the methods aim to remove dead and abnormal sperm and other cells from the sample thereby leaving only normal motile sperm in clean culture medium.

Rarely, the man may be asked to produce another sample that same morning. This happens when the initial sample is of poor quality and it is hoped that a second sample will be better. This is one of the reasons why the man should not leave the center without checking with the IVF laboratory. This is to make sure that there is no problem with the semen sample he produced earlier on.

Progesterone supplementation

It is routine for women who have had GnRHa administration to be given progesterone because they may not produce enough of the hormone themselves during that treatment cycle.

Progesterone is a hormone that is normally produced by the ovaries after ovulation. It helps to increase the thickness of the endometrium and makes it suitable for implantation of the embryo. Production of progesterone continues after implantation and throughout pregnancy.

The fetus and placenta begin to produce progesterone in early pregnancy. Ovarian production of this hormone is not required by 8-12 weeks of pregnancy; the fetus and placenta would have been producing adequate amounts of the hormone by this time.

Progesterone supplementation is started in the evening following egg collection using one of the natural progesterone preparations. A progesterone suppository is inserted into the vagina or rectum from where it is absorbed into the blood stream. The dose varies amongst different practitioners; an example is 200 mg inserted twice a day (in the morning and at night; 12 hours apart).

The patient decides whether she wants to insert the suppository into the vagina or rectum. However, she should not insert it into the vagina on the morning of embryo transfer. The use of progesterone suppositories is continued until the pregnancy test result is available. If negative, she stops inserting the suppositories; the menstrual period should start shortly. If the patient becomes pregnant, she continues with the supplementation until eight weeks of pregnancy.

Another natural progesterone preparation is in the form of an injection that is administered daily. Crinone is a progesterone gel that can also be inserted into the vagina. It is inserted once a day for supplementation after IVF treatment.

Laboratory phase of IVF treatment

On the day of egg collection

A measured volume of the prepared sperm suspension is added to the dish containing the eggs a few hours after the egg collection. The dish is replaced in the incubator.

On the day after the egg collection

The dish is checked in the morning. The eggs that have been fertilized are identified and placed in fresh dishes of culture medium and returned to the incubator. Unfertilized eggs are discarded. The patient is notified of the fertilization result; normally about 40-70% of the eggs should be fertilized. A tentative decision is made on when embryo replacement will be performed.

On the second day after the egg collection

The embryos may be replaced on this day. Depending on the treatment plan and circumstances, it can also be decided to replace the embryos on the third, fourth or fifth day. The dishes are inspected in the morning to find out whether the fertilized eggs have started dividing.

Each fertilized egg is expected to have divided into 2-4 cells by this time. Some embryos may even have more cells than this; say 5-8 cells, on this second day. All the cells are still enclosed by the eggshell (called zona pellucida). When the fertilized egg starts dividing into cells it is called an embryo.

About 60-90% of fertilized eggs should become embryos. Two to four embryos (usually 2-3 embryos, see the next section below) are selected for replacement in the uterus. Any excess embryos that look normal are frozen. Abnormal looking embryos are discarded.

The number of embryos to replace

This is a contentious issue. It is realized that the chance of pregnancy occurring in any particular patient PARTLY depends on the number of transferred embryos. The more the number of embryos that are transferred the greater the chances of conception, all things being equal. However, the incidence of multiple pregnancy also increases with the number of embryos that are replaced.

If one embryo is electively transferred, the pregnancy rate will be about 10-15% and most of the pregnant women will have a single baby. Rarely (less than 1% of cases) will the single embryo split into two to give identical twins.

If two embryos are transferred the pregnancy rate will be roughly 25-30%; about 74% of the pregnant women will have singleton pregnancies while 25% have twin pregnancies and 1% have triplet pregnancies.

If three embryos are transferred the pregnancy rate is slightly higher at 30-35%, and 70% of the women will have singleton pregnancies; up to 24% of pregnancies are twin pregnancies while triplets will be found in about 5%.

The following table attempts to illustrate this concept further. Multiple pregnancy, especially triplet and above, is associated with many complications, major ones being miscarriage and premature delivery.

A compromise, which many centers adopt, is to transfer three embryos generally. Young patients (early to mid twenties) who are deemed suitable may be advised, to have only two embryos replaced. Four embryos may be transferred in exceptional cases, into women above 38 years, especially if they have had previous unsuccessful treatment cycles. Both the patient and the medical team have to decide on how many embryos to transfer but the patient has the final say on this matter. It is very important that the couple give this issue very careful thought before embarking on IVF treatment.

Table 9. The relationship of number of transferred embryos to pregnancy rates

No. of Embryos	Pregnancy rate	No. of Fetuses in 100 Pregnant Women		
		Single	Twin	Triplet or more
1	10-15%	>99%	<1%	Rare
2	25-30%	74%	25%	1%
3	30-35%	70%	24%	5%

Embryo transfer

The couple are given a time to come to the Center for embryo replacement. The woman does not need to be fasting since a general anesthetic will not be given. It is only in a few instances that general anesthesia will be required. Such patients are identified before hand and asked to come in fasting. Depending on the clinical circumstances, some women may be asked to come in with full bladders.

The couple will first have a discussion with the physician and the embryologist. The treatment results up to that point are discussed and the number of embryos for transfer confirmed. If embryos are available for freezing the couple are asked for their consent for this to be done. Only about 1 in 3 couples have enough embryos of good quality to be frozen. Finally, if a video camera is linked to the microscope, the couple can be shown, on the monitor, the embryos that are to be transferred.

Embryo transfer is usually simple and straightforward. It is not a painful procedure. The woman is positioned appropriately and a vaginal speculum inserted so that the cervix ('the mouth of the womb") is seen. The cervical opening is gently wiped with moist cotton wool balls.

At times forceps are applied on the cervix to stabilize it. This will also straighten the angle between the cervical canal and the uterine cavity thereby making embryo transfer easier.

The embryologist then picks up all the embryos to be transferred with a thin polythene tube (catheter) that is attached to a syringe and hands over to the physician. The physician gently inserts the catheter into the uterine cavity through the cervical opening and expels the embryos, with a drop of fluid.

The catheter is then removed and examined under the microscope by the embryologist to ensure that all embryos had been expelled from the catheter. Other instruments are removed from the vagina and the woman left to lie on the examination table for some minutes after which she gets up and goes home.

An adequate supply of the progesterone suppository is provided for her to use during the following 15 days. There does not seem to be much a woman can do to influence the course of events once the embryos have been trans-ferred into the uterus. The most she can be told is to resume her normal activities but avoid doing anything she might later blame herself for doing if she happens not to get pregnant.

Sexual intercourse can be resumed after two days for those who wish to do so. Some couples prefer not to have sex until the results of the treatment are known two weeks later. The woman is asked to come back for a pregnancy test if her periods do not start 14 days after the egg retrieval.

Embryo freezing

Technology is available for freezing embryos. However not all embryos will survive the freezing and thawing process. Furthermore, the pregnancy rate after transfer of frozen-thawed embryos may be less than that following trans-fer of freshly generated embryos.

However, the availability of frozen embryos increases the pregnancy poten-tial of each IVF treatment cycle; from one episode of egg collection, a patient may have 2-3 episodes of embryo replacement. It should be noted that only about 30% of patients would have excess good quality embryos remaining after IVF treatment that are suitable for freezing.

Embryo storage

Frozen embryos can be stored for a long time but moral dilemmas arise the longer they are left unused. This writer recommends that couples should use their stored embryos within 2-5 years.

Options are available for couples who do not want to use their frozen embryos. They include donation to other couples who cannot generate embryos of their own due to one problem or the other. Alternatively, the embryos can be used for research into ways of improving the outcome of assisted conception treatments and prevention of the transfer of genetic diseases. Finally, the couple can ask for the embryos to be destroyed. These options can only be exercised after signed consent is obtained from the couple who generated the embryos.

All couples who have frozen embryos must contact the IVF unit every year to pay the storage fee for the coming year. They also have to sign a form saying that they would like the embryos to be stored for another year. If they fail to do so they have broken their contract with the IVF center regarding storage of the embryos. This implies that the IVF center is legally free to do whatever they believe is ethically justified and the most likely action will be to destroy the embryos.

The regulatory body for IVF and similar treatments in England ordered the destruction of such embryos some years ago. This was carried out amidst publicity and controversy. This author is not advocating any option within the context of this publication except to make patients realize the importance of keeping in touch with the IVF unit if they have embryos that are being stored.

The fate of the transferred embryos

No one knows exactly what happens to the embryos over the ensuing days following their transfer into the uterus. They may remain at the point where they were deposited or may be moved around the uterine cavity by fluid currents, contractions of the endometrium and/or uterine muscle (myometrium).

The fact that some women may have ectopic pregnancy (implantation of the embryo in the fallopian tube) implies that some embryos, at least, may enter the tubes and re-enter the uterine cavity at the normal time of implantation. In the natural situation, an ovulated egg is fertilized in the fallopian tube within a few hours and then moves down the fallopian tube. The embryo reaches the uterine cavity five days later and implants about a day after that. The same might happen to some or all of the embryos that are transferred after IVF.

From the time of embryo transfer, until implantation is complete the embryos are nourished by fluid secreted by glands in the endometrium and maybe fallopian tubes. The embryo implants by hatching through the eggshell (zona pellucida) and burrowing into the endometrium. It then forms the placenta and starts to grow and develop into a recognizable human being.

By the time two weeks have elapsed from the time of embryo transfer the embryo has already started producing a hormone called HCG. This hormone signals to various organ systems in the mother's body alerting them to the presence of a new pregnancy. Human chorionic gonadotropin is what is detected in blood or urine by pregnancy tests.

The pregnancy test

The two-week period of waiting for the pregnancy test is probably the most stressful of the events of IVF treatment. Unfortunately, not much can be done about it. However, good psychological preparation and counseling support can reduce the stress and make the couple cope better with the period of uncertainty.

The patient's urine or blood sample is used for the pregnancy test. The test is rapid and results should be known immediately.

Most times the result is clearly positive or negative. Occasionally, it is equivocal. In this case, the concentration of HCG is measured in that same blood sample and in another blood sample that is withdrawn a week later.

The success rate of IVF

Success following IVF and other assisted conception treatments can be assessed in a number of ways. The most relevant from the patient's perspective is having a clinical pregnancy and a baby. A clinical pregnancy is a pregnancy that is demonstrated to be viable at the first ultrasound scan that is carried out three weeks after a positive pregnancy test.

About 30-50% of women who start each cycle of IVF treatment achieve clinical pregnancies. The success rate depends on several factors some of which are unknown. The known determinants of success include the cause of the infertility, age of the female, the response to ovarian stimulation and semen quality.

The number of embryos generated and transferred, and how good the transferred embryos look are other factors that influence the pregnancy rate. Women who have had prior pregnancies (natural or IVF) have a better chance of falling pregnant with IVF treatment.

Some patients succeed in getting pregnant in the first cycle of treatment. Others may require two or more cycles of treatment to do so. Some women may never become pregnant irrespective of the number of times they have the treatment.

Since some of the pregnancies end in miscarriage or as ectopic pregnancies the proportion of women who will deliver live normal babies will be less than the above figure of 30-50%. The so-called 'take home baby rate' is about 20-40%.

IVF compared to natural pregnancy rates

The IVF pregnancy rates may not appear encouraging initially but it may not be very different from what happens in nature. About 30% of the so-called fertile population succeed in getting pregnant naturally in the first month of trying. The following month the success rate decreases to say 20-25%.

The rate keeps on falling every month until the sixth month when it is 5%. From then onwards only about 5% of couples who have still not achieved pregnancies by then succeed in doing so each month.

Although the IVF pregnancy rate starts relatively low, the rate does not usually fall appreciably with each cycle of treatment unlike what obtains in natural conceptions. Rather, it remains relatively constant. When the proportion of couples who succeed in getting pregnant within one year of trying naturally (about 80%) is compared to that found after four cycles of IVF treatment in one year (about 60-90%) it will be seen that there is not much difference in the rates.

This way of looking at total conceptions within an extended period is called the cumulative pregnancy rate; it has changed the way success at IVF treatment is regarded.

Of course everyone, including the medical team, wants the treatment to succeed and as soon as possible. This is because of the expensive nature of the treatment, the risk of injury during and after the treatment, associated stress and disruption of the couples' routine and work. Attempts are continually being made to improve the success of this and other types of assisted conception treatment.

Negative outcome of IVF treatment

Patients in whom the menstrual period commences beforehand do not need to have the pregnancy test. Such bleeding invariably means that they are not pregnant. If however the bleeding is very scanty and can be described as mere spotting of blood, the test can be performed to clarify issues.

All women with negative outcome (either negative pregnancy test or commencement of menstrual period) are asked to stop using the progesterone supplementation. They are given appointments to come back for review by the physician.

The fact that menstrual periods have not commenced in a female who is on progesterone supplementation after IVF treatment does not necessarily mean that she is pregnant since progesterone can postpone menstrual periods. Menstruation occurs following discontinuation of the medication.

At the next appointment, the concluded IVF treatment cycle is reviewed. An attempt is made to find out why pregnancy did not occur. Decisions are made on whether any future treatment cycle can be modified in any way to improve the chance of successful outcome. Usually, no obvious cause is found for the failed treatment cycle. If embryos were frozen the couple have a choice between using the frozen embryos or accumulating more frozen embryos by having another IVF treatment cycle. The latter option may be chosen in an older woman in whom the remaining period of optimal ovarian function is uncertain. Such women can have many fresh IVF cycles with storage of excess embryos for potential use in future when their ovarian function would have become very poor.

Positive pregnancy test result

Patients who have positive pregnancy test results will continue with the progesterone supplementation as directed. An ultrasound scan is performed 2-3 weeks after the positive pregnancy test. This is to check whether the fetus is alive and growing and the number of fetuses in the uterus.

If the findings are normal, the supplementation is continued for another two weeks. It is the practice of many physicians for the patient to gradually decrease the dose of progesterone in the last week of use. An example is 200 mg twice daily for four days and 200 mg once a day for three days and then stopping the medication on the eighth day. An alternative is to insert a 200 mg suppository once a day during the last week of use.

The timing of ultrasound scans during pregnancy

The age of any pregnancy is conventionally calculated from two weeks before the expected day of fertilization. Thus, women who have had successful IVF treatment are regarded as being four weeks pregnant at the time of the pregnancy test which is normally performed two weeks from the day of egg collection.

It follows that the first ultrasound scan is performed at 6-7 weeks of pregnancy; the use of progesterone supplementation is discontinued on completion of the 8th week of pregnancy. Another ultrasound scan is performed at 12 weeks of pregnancy.

The patient is referred back to her obstetrician for pregnancy care after the 12 week ultrasound scan. It is advisable to have another scan at 19 and 32 weeks of pregnancy. The duration of pregnancy is 40 weeks but women start delivering from two weeks before this time (i.e. 38 weeks) and continue to do so normally until two weeks later (i.e. 42 weeks).

The welfare of IVF babies

Babies delivered as a result of IVF treatment and other assisted conception treatments do not seem to have a congenital malformation rate that is greater than that of the normal population, which is less than 5%. Behaviorally they are similar to other children, although they are loved and pampered a bit more than usual!

Their fathers have been found to show more interest in their daily care more than fathers of babies who were conceived naturally do. There is no evidence at present to show that their development is different from that of other children and young adults. The first IVF baby, who was born in 1978, is now more 26 years old.

Conclusion

In vitro fertilization treatment is complex and some patients initially find it disorienting. Prior preparation by reading about the procedure helps many couples cope with the myriad steps involved. The physicians and nursing staff also provide several information sessions and lectures before hand. This treatment technique has become very successful in recent years. See Appendices VIII-XVI for additional practical information. This chapter was adapted from

Cambridge Guide to Infertility Management and Assisted Reproduction, Cambridge University Press, Cambridge.

10

Intracytoplasmic sperm injection

Introduction

The injection of a single sperm directly into the center of an egg is called intracytoplasmic sperm injection (ICSI). This has now become the treatment of choice for couples with severe male factor problems. Less than 10% of patients fail to achieve fertilization using ICSI. The pregnancy rate following ICSI is similar to that obtained with conventional in vitro fertilization (IVF) treatment for other causes of infertility.

Indications

Intracytoplasmic sperm injection is utilized whenever there is a significant risk of failed fertilization of the eggs using conventional IVF treatment (Table 10). Couples whose eggs were not fertilized by sperm during a previous IVF treatment have an above average risk of having a similar problem in a future IVF treatment. Patients with severe male factor problems constitute another group of patients for whom it is more prudent to perform ICSI rather than IVF.

Antisperm antibodies bind with sperm and interfere with their motion such that the chance of fertilization decreases significantly. The use of ICSI overcomes this impediment and normal fertilization rates are obtained. Some men with azoospermia may still have sperm in their testes. The sperm can be removed directly from the testes or epididymis and used for ICSI treatment. Without ICSI it is difficult to achieve normal fertilization rates with surgically retrieved sperm.

There is a new treatment that is being evaluated for use in treating some groups of infertility patients called in vitro egg maturation. Immature eggs are obtained from the ovary using different techniques. The eggs are incubated in the laboratory for some days to enable them become mature. The mature eggs are then injected with sperm (ICSI), rather than using conventional IVF, to ensure they fertilize.

Table 10. Indications for intracytoplasmic sperm injection

Previous failed fertilization with conventional in vitro fertilization

Moderate-severely abnormal seminal/sperm parameters

Antisperm antibodies

Surgically retrieved sperm

In vitro matured eggs

Conduct of treatment

The conduct of an ICSI treatment cycle is largely similar to that of conventional IVF. Thus, the woman is administered injections to stimulate the growth of several eggs in her ovaries. Ultrasound scan and blood tests are performed to monitor her response to the injections. The eggs are aspirated from the ovaries through the vagina using the ultrasound scanner for guidance.

The only major difference is that with ICSI one sperm is injected directly into each egg. In conventional IVF the eggs are placed in a dish together with several thousand sperm, with the expectation that one sperm will succeed in penetrating and fertilizing each egg. (Normally, the egg prevents entry by other sperm once the first sperm fertilizes it).

Other aspects of the treatment with ICSI including the use of progesterone supplementation, embryo transfer, pregnancy test and ultrasound scanning are similar to those of conventional IVF.

Success rate of ICSI treatment

Factors that influence the outcome of treatment using ICSI, similar to conventional IVF, include the age of the woman producing the eggs, the number of mature eggs available for ICSI, and the number of embryos transferred.

Whilst the overall success of the ICSI treatment is of the order of 30-50% per attempt, it may be higher or lower depending on the particular combination of factors that are present in a specific couple.

Safety of ICSI

Concern has been raised in certain quarters regarding the safety of ICSI. This concern is instinctive given the fact that ICSI is one of the more radical advanced reproductive technologies. This is a controversial area and there is presently no categorical information to settle the matter.

It does not appear that ICSI in itself gives rise to problems in the children so conceived. Men with severe male factor infertility problems tend to have a higher incidence of genetic problems. It follows that the children of such men whether conceived by ICSI, IVF or any other assisted conception method will inherit some of those genetic problems. However, looking at population statistics it does not appear that the incidence of congenital malformation in these children is greater than that found in children who are conceived naturally. Genetic tests are now available for men with severe male factor infertility problems.

Conclusion

The ability to achieve normal fertilization rates through the use of ICSI has forever changed the management of male factor infertility. It has also improved the expectation of couples with male factor problems; previously their only recourse was to use donor sperm for infertility treatment, adopt or lead a child free existence. More information is still being generated about ICSI treatment including safety issues. There is however, no doubt that the availability of ICSI has made it possible for many more men to have offspring who are genetically related to them than would have been possible in previous years.

11

Frozen embryo replacement

Introduction

Frozen embryo replacement (FER) has been used for several years in treating infertile couples. Several thousand healthy babies have now been born worldwide following FER. Any good quality embryo that remains following in vitro fertilization (IVF) treatment can be frozen for potential transfer in a future treatment cycle. Embryo thawing followed by transfer is performed when the woman's endometrium is at the right phase of the menstrual cycle.

Management of the FER treatment cycle

The frozen embryo replacement cycle is relatively non-invasive compared to an egg retrieval cycle. The embryos can be replaced either in a natural cycle or in a controlled cycle. In a controlled cycle, a gonadotropin releasing hormone agonist is first administered to suppress the pituitary gland.

Estrogen tablets are administered daily to prepare the endometrium for implantation as an alternative to the natural changes occurring in the endometrium in a spontaneous ovulatory cycle (see Appendix XVII).

The development of the endometrium is monitored by ultrasound scanning; approximately four episodes of scanning or less will be required. Either when ovulation has occurred, or when the endometrium is thick enough, the embryos can be thawed for replacement.

Thawing of the embryos

The embryologist will thaw the embryos so that the stage of the embryos corresponds to the replacement cycle. The exact timing will depend upon the stage at which the embryos were frozen.

Not all embryos survive the freezing, storage and thawing process. On the morning of the embryo transfer, the embryologist will assess the embryos to see if they are suitable for transfer.

The embryo transfer

For this procedure, a fine tube (catheter) containing the embryos is passed through the cervix. The embryos are gently ejected into the cavity of the uterus in a minute amount of culture medium. This technique does not normally require sedation, and is not painful.

After the embryo transfer

Natural progesterone suppositories will be provided for insertion into the rectum or vagina 2-3 times daily. The hormone is absorbed from these sites to support the lining of the uterus. A pregnancy test is carried out 12 days after the embryo transfer.

The success rate of FER

The success rate using frozen thawed embryos is between 10-50% or more, depending on the individual patient's characteristics as described in previous chapters.

Conclusion

The ability to freeze embryos has extended the potentials of IVF treatment. Excess embryos can be frozen for possible use in future. Even if a woman becomes pregnant following an initial IVF treatment, she can still have further pregnancies established with the frozen embryos. This will avoid repeating fresh IVF treatment cycles, which are more expensive and traumatic than FER. The ability to freeze embryos can also permit physicians to manage certain complications by deferring embryo transfer and freezing the embryos. Such complications include ovarian hyperstimulation syndrome (OHSS). Following recovery from OHSS, the embryos are transferred in an FER cycle.

Finally, donated eggs can be fertilized and frozen as embryos for quarantine. After six months the egg donor is retested for human immunodeficiency virus infection. If the test is negative the embryos can then be transferred into the recipient.

12

Egg donation

Introduction

Egg donation is offered by many infertility treatment programs for certain groups of patients. It is a complex process that involves not only medical and surgical interventions but counseling, psychological and legal preparation and oversight. These processes will ensure that the interests and welfare of all parties to the treatment are safeguarded.

This chapter contains information that provides the basis for the treatment as offered at Junaelo Institute of Reproductive Medicine. It explains in clear terms most of what will be involved. It is very important that all individuals who are involved in this treatment understand the procedures and implication of the whole treatment.

Indications for egg donation

Egg donation is required for women who are unable to use their own eggs for procreation. This includes women with:

- Ovarian failure.

- Surgical castration (removal of the ovaries).

- Inheritable (genetic) disease that is not desirable to be passed unto the next generation (children).

- Failed repeated attempts at in vitro fertilization (IVF) treatment.

- Inaccessible ovaries.
- Poor response to ovarian stimulation.
- Persistently poor outcome of infertility treatment.
- Older woman (above 42 years).

Types of donors

There are two types of donors. An "anonymous egg donor" is one of whom the recipient is not aware of her identity. If the recipient knows who donated the eggs the donor is said to be "known".

Source of donors

Donors come from diverse sources such as the following:

- A friend or relative of the recipient.
- An infertile woman who wishes to donate her eggs in order to reduce the cost of her treatment.
- The donor can be recruited by the recipient through advertisement in newspapers and other media or through egg donor agencies.
- The donor may be recruited by the infertility treatment facility itself.

Donor's age and other characteristics

It is desirable that the donor be in her twenties and not more than 30 years of age. It is well known that the older a woman is the less is the pregnancy potential of her eggs. There is also an increasing incidence of abnormal chromosomes in the eggs and miscarriage especially if the donor is above 30 years old. If however, a younger donor cannot be found donors up to the age of 35 years may be accepted; the recipient should be counseled on having prenatal diagnostic tests for Down's syndrome and other anomalies that can be screened for, when she becomes pregnant.

The donor may be married or unmarried. She can also have her own children or may not have had any pregnancies. The donor should be aware of the fact that she cannot lay any claim on the retrieved eggs or resulting embryos and children, even if she subsequently becomes infertile.

Screening

To ensure that the egg donation process is safe for both donor and recipient complete evaluation of the three individuals who will be involved in the treatment is performed. This is a multicomponent/multidimensional evaluation process that involves medical, laboratory and psychological testing.

Donor screening

1. Medical history.

2. Genetic history.

3. Other information of possible interest to resulting progeny and anonymous recipients:

   a. Age

   b. Height

   c. Weight

   d. Eye color

   e. Hair color

   f. Skin color

   g. Religion

   h. Nationality of donor, her parents and grandparents.

   i. Ethnicity of donor, donor's parents and grandparents.

   j. Country of birth of donor, donor's parents and grandparents.

   k. Highest educational level.

   l. Occupation.

   m. Marital status.

   n. Number of children.

o. Interests (hobbies, sports etc).

p. Reason for donating eggs.

4. Psychological evaluation by means of history and sessions with the counselor/psychologist.

5. Physical examination.

6. Ultrasound scan.

7. Laboratory tests:

   a. Pap smear.

   b. Blood group, Rhesus type and antibody screen.

   c. Complete blood count.

   d. Complete metabolic panel.

   e. Karyotyping (Checking for chromosome number and shape).

   f. Menstrual cycle Day 3 test for follicle stimulating hormone (FSH), luteinizing hormone (LH), Prolactin and Estradiol.

8. Infectious screen using the following tests:

   a. HIV 1 & 2 (Human Immunodeficiency Virus)

   b. HBsAg (Hepatitis B surface Antigen)

   c. HBcAb (Hepatitis B core Antibody)

   d. Hepatitis C Antibody

   e. HTLV-1 antibodies

   f. Tests (RPR, VDRL) for Syphilis

   g. CMV IgM antibody (Cytomegalovirus)

   h. Cervical cultures

   i. Gonorrhea

   j. Chlamydia

   k. Mycoplasma/Ureaplasma

l. Herpes simplex virus (by taking a cervical and vaginal swab at the time of egg collection).

m. Other tests as indicated

    i. Sickle cell disease/anemia (e.g. Africans, African Americans)

    ii. Thalassemia (Mediterranean Europeans or Asians)

    iii. Tay-Sachs disease (e.g. Ashkenazi Jews)

    iv. Canavan's disease (e.g. Ashkenazi Jews)

    v. Cystic fibrosis (e.g. Caucasians, but all ethnic groups should ideally have the test)

    vi. Factor V Leiden mutation

9. Donor to sign a lifestyle declaration document (Appendix XIX).

See Appendices XX-XXII for further details of donor screening.

Recipient screening

1. History and Physical Examination.

2. Uterine cavity evaluation by sonohysterography or hysterosalpingography.

3. Mock embryo transfer.

4. +/- Trial cycle with estrogens and progesterone to determine whether the endometrium will respond to these hormones in the definitive cycle; this is optional but the patient decides.

5. Endometrial biopsy during the trial cycle

6. Evaluation by a Maternal Fetal Medicine specialist (in older aged women and those with medical conditions that may be worsened by pregnancy).

7. Counseling and psychological evaluation.

8. Laboratory tests:

a. Pap smear.

b. Blood group, Rhesus type and antibody screen.

c. Complete blood count.

d. Complete metabolic panel.

e. Rubella antibody level (to verify immunity to rubella a.k.a. German measles).

f. Karyotyping (checking for chromosome number and shape).

g. Urinalysis and culture.

h. +/- EKG (electrocardiogram).

i. +/- Chest X-Ray.

j. +/- Mammogram.

k. +/- Cholesterol and lipid profile.

l. +/- Glucose tolerance test (screens for diabetes mellitus)

m. +/- Thyroid function test.

9. Infectious screen using the following tests:

a. HIV 1 & 2 (Human Immunodeficiency Virus).

b. HBsAg (Hepatitis B surface Antigen).

c. HBcAb (Hepatitis B core Antibody).

d. Hepatitis C Antibody.

e. HTLV-1 antibodies.

f. Tests (RPR, VDRL) for Syphilis

g. CMV IgM antibody (Cytomegalovirus).

h. Cervical cultures.

i. Gonorrhea.

j. Chlamydia.

k. Mycoplasma/Ureaplasma.

l. Other tests as indicated:

   i. Sickle cell disease/anemia (e.g. Africans, African Americans)

   ii. Thalassemia (Mediterranean Europeans or Asians)

   iii. Tay-Sachs disease (e.g. Ashkenazi Jews)

   iv. Canavan's disease (e.g. Ashkenazi Jews)

   v. Cystic fibrosis (e.g. Caucasians, but ideally all ethnic groups should have the test)

   vi. Factor V Leiden mutation

Husband screening

1. Semen analysis

2. Sperm longevity test for couples who will have conventional IVF treatment. The semen sample is processed and incubated for 48 hours to determine how long the sperm can survive.

3. Sperm freezing and test thaw for semen backup. This is optional although it is encouraged in case the man is unable to produce a semen sample on the day of egg retrieval.

4. Infectious screen using the following tests:

   a. HIV 1 & 2 (Human Immunodeficiency Virus).

   b. HBsAg (Hepatitis B surface Antigen).

   c. HBcAb (Hepatitis B core Antibody).

   d. Hepatitis C Antibody.

   e. Tests (RPR, VDRL) for Syphilis.

Psychological evaluation and counseling

The psychological results of donating eggs may not be predictable in all cases. The proposed donor must have a high degree of conviction of her motives of becoming a donor. The counselor will evaluate both donor and recipient. Psychosocial, ethical and legal issues surrounding egg donation will be examined with both women; long and short term implications will also be identified and discussed.

Folic acid supplementation

Both the donor and the recipient should take folic acid tablets at a dose of 0.4 mg once a day starting before ovarian stimulation is commenced. After the egg retrieval the donor may discontinue taking the vitamin while the recipient continues hers. If the recipient becomes pregnant she should continue taking folic acid tablets until 8 weeks of pregnancy at which time she can change to taking a prenatal vitamin preparation that contains a similar amount of folic acid.

Folic acid supplementation that was started before conception and continued for the first three months of pregnancy has been shown to reduce the fetal risk of developing spina bifida ("hole in the spine") and other neural tube defects.

Hormonal preparation of the donor and egg retrieval

Pre-treatment of the donor with oral contraceptive pills or progestin medication is carried out. This helps quieting the ovary and synchronize the menstrual cycle to enable the menstrual period occur at the required time.

A long acting gonadotropin releasing hormone agonist (GnRHa) such as Zoladex or Lupron is administered some days before the expected menstrual period or following commencement of the menses. One depot injection of this medication lasts for 28 days approximately. Alternatively, shorter acting brands can be administered by daily injection (Lupron) or sniffing into the nose (Synarel [Nafarelin]).

The GnRHa medications lead to temporary suppression of the pituitary gland (found in the brain) and the ovaries. This prevents the pituitary from interfering with the development of the eggs in the ovaries and causing premature ovulation.

An ultrasound scan and blood tests for estrogen, FSH and LH are performed 10-14 days after administering the GnRHa. The results of these tests will show whether the pituitary gland has been suppressed. The ultrasound scan will also confirm that no ovarian cyst has formed.

Daily injections of FSH (various brands) are then started and given for 10-14 days. This will stimulate the development of several follicles in both ovaries. The development of the follicles is monitored using ultrasound scans and measuring the levels of estradiol and other hormones in blood.

When the size of the follicles reaches a certain range an injection of human chorionic gonadotropin (HCG) is administered. HCG induces final maturation of the eggs, each of which is contained in a follicle.

Retrieval of the eggs is performed about 36 hours after the HCG injection. Intravenous medications are administered for pain relief and sedation to abolish discomfort during the procedure. These medications are short-acting and the patient is able to go home 1-2 hours later. Using ultrasound guidance a hollow needle is used to puncture the top of the vagina then the ovaries and drain as many of the follicles in the ovaries as possible. As the follicles are drained the egg tends to detach from it's attachment to the wall of the follicle and is aspirated by the needle into sterile tubes.

The laboratory scientist identifies the eggs in the follicular aspirates and transfer's them into culture dishes that are placed in the incubator. Later on these eggs will be fertilized with the recipient's husband's sperm.

Post retrieval care of the donor

Analgesics (pain killers) and antibiotics are administered to the donor afterwards and she is discharged home. This marks the end of participation of the egg donor in the treatment cycle. However, she is not ignored since she may develop complications following the treatment and these may manifest several days after the retrieval. The donor is advised to rest for about two weeks and avoid vigorous exercise.

There is a risk that some eggs may remain in her pelvis or ovulated from the ovaries after the retrieval. This could lead to pregnancy and possibly high order multiple pregnancy if she has unprotected sexual intercourse. She is therefore advised to either abstain from sex for two weeks or use condoms. In the normal course of events she will have a menstrual period about 10-16 days after the egg retrieval.

Complications that may be experienced by the donor

Several complications and side effects can occur during and after treatment. These include poor ovarian response, ovarian hyperstimulation syndrome, infection, trauma to pelvic organs, bleeding from pelvic organs, ectopic pregnancy, ovarian torsion, initial menopause-type symptoms, multiple pregnancy, failed fertilization, poor embryo development and failed treatment. This is not an exhaustive list. Ovarian stimulation is rarely associated with subsequent development of ovarian tumors but this is controversial.

The needle used for the egg retrieval procedure may cause injury to internal organs such as the bladder, ureters, uterus and bowel. There may be hemorrhage from the ovaries, vagina or the pelvic blood vessels. There is also a risk of infection. Some patients may have to be admitted to hospital for observation or surgery and repair of the injured organs.

The medications used for conscious sedation can cause various drugs reactions including allergic reactions, heart rate abnormalities, low or high blood pressure and depression of the breathing.

There may be a failure to retrieve eggs. There are other unforeseen problems that may arise leading to loss of eggs or embryos such as prolonged power failure and equipment breakdown.

Ovarian hyperstimulation syndrome can arise several days after egg retrieval. The ovaries enlarge and secrete a large amount of fluid into the abdominal cavity. The fluid can accumulate around the lungs and heart in severe cases. The patient develops abdominal discomfort and distension. She gains weight rapidly. Urine output may decrease or stop altogether. Several other complications can arise in patients with this syndrome and some patients may die.

The mild-moderate type of ovarian hyperstimulation syndrome occurs in about 25% of women who have ovarian stimulation for IVF treatment. These women are managed by bed rest at home, use of analgesics, increased intake of oral fluid and protein in the diet. The severe variety occurs in about 1% of women. This is usually managed by hospital admission and supportive care with intravenous fluids and other measures. All varieties of this syndrome are self-limiting and gradually resolve.

Hormonal preparation of the egg recipient

The recipient's menstrual cycle is synchronized with that of her egg donor so that hormonal preparation of both women can be conducted at the same time. It may be necessary for the recipient to be pre-treated with oral contraceptives or progestins prior to the administration of the GnRHa (e.g. Nafarelin, Lupron, and Zoladex). Following confirmation of pituitary suppression and ovarian quiescence by ultrasound scan and hormone blood tests, preparation of the lining of the womb (endometrium) for receipt of the embryos is commenced.

This is achieved by administering estrogen preparations to the recipient. Administration can be achieved with tablets, injections or skin patches. An example is estradiol tablet that is administered at a dose of 2 mg twice a day for one week after which the frequency is increased to three times a day.

Following retrieval of eggs from the donor the recipient adds progesterone to the medications she is taking. Progesterone helps with the final preparation of the endometrium for implantation of the embryo. Following conception, estrogen and progesterone continue to support further growth and development of the endometrium which is now called the decidua of pregnancy.

A common way of administering progesterone is as suppositories that are inserted into the vagina twice a day. Progesterone can also be given as a daily intramuscular injection.

Both methods of administration are equally efficacious but the injection is much more expensive than progesterone suppositories and painful to administer.

Both estradiol and progesterone administration are continued after the embryo transfer until a pregnancy test is performed about two weeks later. If the result is negative the medications are stopped and menses occurs soon afterwards. Some women who are not pregnant will even start having their menstrual period while they are still taking these medications. They should stop the medications once menstrual bleeding is established. If the pregnancy test is positive both estrogen and progesterone administration is continued until 12 weeks of pregnancy.

Monitoring of endometrial preparation

Ultrasound scans are carried out at various stages of the recipient's endometrial preparation. It is performed about 10-14 days after administering the GnRHa to confirm pituitary suppression. It will also demonstrate that the endometirium is thin (usually less than 5 mm in thickness) and that there are no ovarian cysts.

Ultrasound scanning is subsequently repeated at intervals during administration of estrogen and progesterone. This will document continued endometrial development until the endometirium is judged suitable for embryo transfer.

If endometrial development is found to be inadequate the embryos are frozen and another cycle of endometrial preparation commenced after inducing withdrawal bleeding.

Fertilization of the eggs

The recipient's partner produces a semen sample by masturbation on the day of egg retrieval. The semen is processed to select out only the live, motile and normal looking sperm. The prepared sperm sample is placed in a labeled tube and kept in the incubator until required.

The eggs will be fertilized using one of two techniques depending on the husband's semen quality. If a previous semen analysis demonstrated the sperm quality to be normal conventional IVF treatment will be performed. However, there is always a risk of failed fertilization with conventional IVF techniques irrespective of how normal the sperm appear to be. If the sperm quality is abnormal intracytoplasmic sperm injection (ICSI) is carried out to prevent a total failure of fertilization.

Conventional IVF treatment is performed by adding a measured volume of the prepared sperm sample to the dish that contains the retrieved eggs. The dish is then replaced in the incubator and checked the following morning to find out which eggs fertilized normally. It is hoped that at least 50% of the eggs will be fertilized. The fertilized eggs are placed in fresh culture dishes and replaced in the incubator.

Intracytoplasmic sperm injection is performed by injecting a single sperm into each mature egg. Not all the retrieved eggs will be mature and suitable for injection. About 50% or more of the injected eggs fertilize normally.

Embryo development and transfer

About 70-90% of fertilized eggs develop into embryos and divide into increasingly smaller cells (blastomeres) which are retained within the 'egg shell' or zona pellucida. The embryos are usually ready for transfer into the recipient's uterus by the second or third day following egg retrieval.

The selected number of embryos, usually not more than three, is transferred into the uterus 2-6 days following the egg retrieval. This does not require anesthesia and is quick. A speculum is placed in the vagina to allow visualization of the cervix. The cervix is gently cleansed several times with sterile cotton wool balls that are soaked in normal saline solution. A small amount of the culture medium is then used to wipe the cervix further.

The embryos are loaded into a thin polythene tube that is attached to a syringe. The catheter is then introduced into the uterine cavity through the cervix and the embryos deposited there by depressing the plunger of the syringe. The catheter is gently removed and examined under the microscope to ensure that there is no embryo remaining in the catheter.

The speculum and other instruments are then removed followed by tilting the bed on which the patient is lying slightly head down. The woman is observed for some minutes before being discharged home.

Fresh versus frozen embryo transfer

There has been concern about a persisting risk of transferring infection to the recipient through the donor eggs even after the donor tests negative for infections such as HIV and Hepatitis B or C. This is because some donors who acquire these infections may not show evidence of infection on blood testing until up to six months afterwards.

In order to avoid this occurrence, which so far does not seem to have happened, some authorities have proposed that all embryos are frozen for at least six months. This allows retesting of the donor for the same infections; if the test results are negative at the end of this quarantine period embryo transfer can then proceed.

The required number of embryos is thawed and transferred after preparing the recipient's endometrium as already described. In this case estradiol is administered for 14 days followed by addition of progesterone to the drug regimen and embryo transfer.

Treatment with thawed frozen embryos following egg donation as described above is an accepted treatment strategy and is performed in some infertility programs. However it is associated with a lower pregnancy rate when compared to the transfer of fresh (non-frozen-thawed) embryos. The ultimate decision should be made by the recipient after considering all aspects of the debate.

Following embryo transfer

Although there may be no hard scientific evidence to support this patients are normally told after embryo transfer to have bed-rest at home for two days. After this they should generally take things easy for two weeks and abstain from sexual intercourse. A more realistic advice is for the patient not to do anything that she may regret if the pregnancy test result happens to be negative afterwards.

Success rate

Egg donation is associated with a higher pregnancy rate in the recipient than is obtained using her eggs. Rates of 35-50% or higher may be obtained in each treatment cycle. However, there is no guarantee that pregnancy will occur in a first or any specific treatment cycle. Some women will only get pregnant after several cycles of treatment. This fact has to borne in mind, when contemplating treatment, due to the high costs involved.

Excess embryos and cryostorage

Excess embryos are normally frozen for potential use to generate more pregnancies in future. If the recipient becomes pregnant with the first batch of transferred embryos she can use embryos from the frozen stored batch later on if she wants more pregnancies. This avoids having to go through another elaborate cycle of egg donation.

Disposal of unwanted frozen embryos

If the recipient decides not to use any more of the embryos still in frozen storage she may wish them to be thawed and discarded, donated to a needy couple, used for research or kept in storage indefinitely. Many programs have stipulations that stored embryos should be used within five years or disposed.

Complications in the recipient

Problems that may be experienced by the recipient include drug side effects of estrogen such as nausea, vomiting, headache, and formation of clots in the lower limb blood vessels. These clots may lead to stroke, heart attack or shortness of breath. Progesterone may cause drowsiness and breast tenderness. Pelvic infection can happen if vaginal micro-organisms gain access to the uterine cavity, fallopian tubes and pelvis.

The most important complication seems to be that of multiple pregnancy. Transfer of more than one embryo is often required to improve the chance of conception. However, if more than one embryo succeeds in implanting this may lead to multiple pregnancy. Although twin pregnancy increases the risks associated with singleton pregnancies triplet and higher order multiple pregnancies are associated with a pronounced increase in the risk of further complications such as miscarriage, preterm labor and delivery.

As already discussed above, no amount of screening can generate a 100% assurance that infections and other diseases cannot be transferred from the donor to the recipient. Infection is always a possibility following tissue donation. There is also a possibility that there is an unknown infection in the donor that has not been discovered by scientists and has no screening test.

The risk of infection exists irrespective of whether the donor is known or anonymous. Recipients should be particularly careful about waiving full screening of relatives or friends who want to be their donors. These acquaintances still have the full potential for infection as compared to anonymous donors.

Financial arrangements

The recipient normally compensates the donor for her time, inconvenience and discomfort by paying her a pre-agreed sum of money once the eggs have been donated. The money is held in escrow by the fertility center or attorney before treatment starts to hold in trust for the donor. If the treatment is completed to the point of egg retrieval the amount is released in full to the donor. If however the donor unilaterally cancels the treatment she is not given this amount. Prorated payments may be made if the cycle is cancelled due to no fault of the donor but this will not exceed 20% of the pre-agreed sum for egg donation. Compensation of the donor is not regarded as payment for her eggs.

The recipient is financially responsible for the management of any medical complications, such as bleeding, infection and OHSS, that may arise in the donor as a result of the treatment.

Ownership of the eggs and embryos

Once the eggs are retrieved from the donor they are regarded as belonging to the recipient. Ownership extends to any resulting embryos and the recipient is solely responsible for the disposition of the embryos.

Offspring

The offspring generated from the donor eggs are regarded as the recipient's children. The egg donor does not have any parenting responsibilities, rights or liability to the offspring or to the recipient couple even if the egg donor and the embryo recipient are related. The donor cannot lay any claim on these off-spring. The egg donor cannot get involved in the rearing of the children unless invited by the recipient through a separately executed contractual agreement. The recipient couple is fully responsible for any and all offspring, regardless of the outcome of the pregnancy.

Anonymity

Except for the case of known donors, the identity of the donor or recipient will not be revealed to any of the two women. The donor will not be given any information on the fate of the eggs, fertilization rate, embryo disposition, pregnancy, pregnancy outcome and resulting children.

In anonymous donation, the donor profile, minus identifying information, will be made available to the recipient if she becomes pregnant from the use of the donor eggs. Despite this no one can guarantee against an accidental disclosure of confidential information on any of both parties to one or both of them.

There is also no prediction of the direction of future legislation and any future requirements regarding the disclosure of identifying information to the donor, recipient, progeny, heirs or any other interested party.

Non-identifying information on the treatment cycle characteristics may be provided to government associated bodies such as the Centers for Disease Control as part of their facility regulatory functions.

Financial responsibility

The recipient couple is fully responsible for all costs incurred as part of the egg donation exercise. These are rarely covered by insurance plans. The couple should seek early written clarification from their insurance carrier.

All financial obligations should be discharged before the treatment is commenced; the recipient couple should make full payment of the estimated cost. It is however, impossible to give an exact cost estimate for the procedure and minor adjustments to the costs may become necessary during the treatment.

These costs will be the full responsibility of the recipient couple who should make the payment immediately the charge is generated. The fertility center has no responsibility to pay for any medical expense that arises as a result of egg donation.

Pregnancy care

The recipient will be referred back to her referring Obstetrician for prenatal care and delivery. The Institute may provide prenatal care and delivery services to pregnant women who request the service and were not referred to the Institute by their Gynecologist.

Conclusion

This account of egg donation will assist decision making by prospective egg donors and recipients. It will also help the individuals to understand and follow the progress of their treatment. It helps them understand their obligations and rights. However, this should not be regarded as an exhaustive account and secondary sources of information should be accessed. Furthermore, the information provided here is continuously updated. Finally, aspects of egg donation, similar to the rest of assisted reproduction technology, are continuously evolving. Practices may change without warning or explanation but will be provided in good fate.

13

Undesirable aspects and complications of infertility management

Introduction

Infertility complicates people's lives; most couples do not seriously consider the possibility of infertility when starting their life together. On the way to achieving pregnancy, several couples may have unpleasant experiences. Most importantly there are several potential complications that may occur during infertility management. Some of these complications may affect the couple as a unit. However, the most serious complications affect the women.

Undesirable aspects of infertility treatment

Expense

Infertility evaluation and treatment are generally expensive, and may not be covered by several government sponsored healthcare delivery programs. Medical insurance plans also do not provide funding for most treatments that have anything to do with infertility. This means that many couples have to directly pay for some or most of the required investigations and treatments. This severely drains the financial resources of infertile couples and some may borrow money to fund such projects.

Strain and stress

Infertility management also imposes a strain on the physical and mental state of couples. They are often required to make several visits to the hospital or physician's office. The requirement for frequent visits increases during advanced reproductive therapy. This disrupts their work routine and special arrangements, including annual leave, may be required.

Impingement of sexual function

The couple's sexual life takes further beating as the man is often required to produce semen samples on demand and in unfamiliar environments. Some men may develop impotence or inability to ejaculate in such situations. The couple's normal rhythm of sexual activity is often disturbed. This is because they may be required to abstain from sexual intercourse at certain times. At other times they may be required to have sex at specific days or time of the day.

Invasive procedures

During advanced reproductive therapy the woman is administered several injections, some of them on a daily basis. These injections may be painful. Several blood samples are usually withdrawn for different tests.

Many of the female investigations such transvaginal ultrasound scans, endometrial biopsy and hysterosalpingogram are not comfortable. Although they may be regarded as being necessary, they are still another invasion of the woman's privacy. Infertile couples are forced by circumstances to put up with a lot of discomfort and disruption of their lives. They do this often with the hope that pregnancy would eventually be achieved thereby rewarding their stoicism and perseverance.

Drug side effects

Minor side effects of administered drugs and hormones include headaches. Some of the medications may need to be administered through the nasal route by sniffing. This may lead to nasal stuffiness and discharge due to irritation of the mucous lining of the nose. There may be allergic reactions to some of the injections.

Other injections may be very painful. Women who are being administered gonadotropin releasing hormone agonists commonly report menopause-type symptoms such as hot flashes.

Cycle cancellation

Some in vitro fertilization (IVF) treatment cycles may be canceled prior to the stage of egg collection. The incidence varies but up to 10-15% of treatment cycles may be canceled. This is usually due to poor response to the ovarian stimulation with the number of developing follicles being less than three.

Occasionally cycle cancellation may be due to a very excessive response. This is called ovarian hyperstimulation syndrome and could become life threatening if HCG is administered. Several options for the prevention and management of this condition are discussed in Chapter 9.

The pituitary gland may release luteinizing hormone (LH) prematurely during advanced reproductive therapy. Such premature surging of LH production by the pituitary gland used to be a common cause of cycle cancellation. However, this is quite uncommon nowadays in treatment cycles that incorporate the use of gonadotropin releasing hormone agonists or antagonists. Both agonists and antagonists suppress pituitary function, preventing the release of LH.

Problems following transvaginal egg retrieval

Egg collection during IVF treatment is most commonly performed by needle aspiration of the ovarian follicles through the vagina. Strong pain relieving medications are given during the procedure. Afterwards some women may experience "period-type cramps" for 1-2 days.

There may be slight bleeding from the area of the vagina that was punctured with the needle during egg collection. The bleeding is usually self limiting and quickly subsides. At times the bleeding may be heavy. Blood vessels in the pelvis can also be punctured during egg collection.

Bowel loops can be perforated with the egg retrieval needle but this may avoided by using a careful technique. Often bowel loops can be seen in the pelvis using the ultrasound probe. Such bowel loops are avoided by maneuvering the probe away from that area.

Pelvic infection can happen after egg collection. Although the vagina is cleansed before the procedure, the vagina is not sterile. Microorganisms that are "normal" inhabitants of the vagina can cause infection if they get transported into the pelvis through the needle. The risk of infection following transvaginal egg collection is low with a rate of 0.58% being quoted by some researchers.

Lack of fertilization

During IVF treatment the partner's sperm is added to a dish containing the woman's eggs. These sperm subsequently fertilize about 40-70% of the eggs. However, occasionally none of the eggs will be fertilized. Fertilization failure can be due to defects in the sperm. It can also be due to abnormal eggs.

Multiple pregnancies

The incidence of multiple pregnancy is high following advanced reproductive therapy. This is because many embryos are commonly produced with these treatments. It is believed that allowing many embryos to try to implant will improve the chances of at least one embryo implanting successfully. This belief is however being challenged now by the good results that are being obtained when only one embryo is transferred into the uterus.

There is therefore a move to the replacement of fewer embryos during IVF treatment. Stimulation of the development of several follicles during intrauterine insemination is also being discouraged.

Multiple pregnancy is accompanied by several risks such as an increased incidence of miscarriage, maternal disease and preterm delivery. These threaten the pregnancy itself, the health of the woman and the lives of the children born afterwards.

Ectopic pregnancy

This is more common after advanced reproductive therapy than in the normal population. The incidence of ectopic pregnancy is 3% after IVF treatment. The reason for this higher incidence is unknown at present. There is a chance that infertile women have a higher chance of having disorders of the fallopian tube than the general population. These will lead to a higher chance of developing ectopic pregnancies in these women. It is also possible that the infertility treatment itself exposes the women to this higher risk. Preventive healthcare has a lot to offer in this area.

Miscarriage

The incidence of miscarriage after IVF treatment is 25%. This rate does not seem to be higher than that of the general population. However, it is possible that infertility patients may have a slightly higher risk of miscarriage than other women.

A link with cancer?

Some researchers have warned of a possible link between ovarian stimulation and a later development of ovarian cancer. However, the evidence for this is not strong. Therefore, this has been a controversial issue for many years. The results of several studies have not supported this assertion. More research is being conducted to determine the truth in this matter. For now the evidence points to the fact that most women who have ovarian stimulation do not develop cancer.

Conclusion

The management of infertility is fraught with several problems. These may prolong the infertile state or lead to the development of complications even after achievement of pregnancy. A careful and compassionate approach to the infertile couple will help reduce the risk of these problems.

Acronyms in infertility management

Acronym	Meaning
AIH	Artificial insemination (with) husband (sperm)
ART	Assisted reproduction (reproductive) technology
ASA	Antisperm antibodies
BBT	Basal body temperature (monitoring)
CASA	Computer assisted semen analysis
CBAVD	Congenital bilateral absence of the vas deferens
CC	Clomiphene citrate
CCT	Clomiphene challenge test
CCCT	Clomiphene citrate challenge test
COH	Controlled ovarian hyperstimulation
COS	Controlled ovarian stimulation
DES	Diethylstilbestrol
DHEAS	Dehydroepiandrosterone sulfate
DI	Donor insemination (used to be called AID [artificial insemination donor] until the advent of AIDS)

Acronym	Meaning
DIFI	Direct intrafollicular insemination
DIPI	Direct intraperitoneal insemination
E1	Estrone
E2	17 ß-Estradiol or oestrogen
E3	Estriol
EDD	Estimated date of delivery
ELSI	Elongated spermatid injection
ET	Embryo transfer
FER	Frozen embryo replacement
FET	Frozen embryo transfer
FSH	Follicle stimulating hormone
GIFT	Gamete intrafallopian transfer
GnRH	Gonadotropin releasing hormone
GnRHa	Gonadotropin releasing hormone analogue (or agonist)
GV	Germinal vesicle (egg)
HCG	Human chorionic gonadotropin
HIC-IVF	High insemination concentration in vitro fertilization
HMG	Human menopausal gonadotropin
HOST	Hypo-osmotic swelling test
HPF	High power field
HRT	Hormone replacement therapy

Acronym	Meaning
HSG	Hysterosalpingogram, hysterosalpingograph, hysterosalpingography
IBT	Immunobead test
ICI	Intracervical insemination
ICSI	Intracytoplasmic sperm injection
IM	Intramuscular (injection)
IPI	Intraperitoneal insemination
ITI	Intratubal insemination
IUCD	Intrauterine contraceptive device
IUI	Intrauterine insemination
IV	Intravenous (injection or infusion)
IVC	Intravaginal culture
IVF	In vitro fertilization
Lap & Dye	Laparoscopy and dye test
LH	Luteinizing hormone
LPD	Luteal phase defect
LUF	Luteinized unruptured follicle (syndrome)
MAF	Micro assisted fertilization
MAR test	Mixed antiglobulin reaction test
MESA	Microepididymal sperm aspiration
MFT	Male fertility test (semen analysis)
MRI	Magnetic resonance imaging

Acronym	Meaning
μIVF	Microdrop in vitro fertilization
OC	Oral contraceptive
OCC	Oocyte cumulus complex
OD	Oocyte donation (oocyte donor)
OHSS	Ovarian hyperstimulation syndrome
OPU	Ovum pick-up
OR	Oocyte recipient
P4	Progesterone
PCO	Polycystic ovaries
PCOD	Polycystic ovary disease
PCOS	Polycystic ovary syndrome
PCT	Post coital test
PESA	Percutaneous epididymal sperm aspiration
PGD	Pre-implantation genetic diagnosis
PID	Pelvic inflammatory disease
POF	Premature ovarian failure
ProST	Pronuclear stage transfer
PZD	Partial zona dissection
ROS	Reactive oxygen species
ROSI	Round spermatid injection
ROSNI	Microinjection of round spermatid nuclei into oocytes
RPL	Recurrent pregnancy loss

Acronym	Meaning
SA	Semen analysis
SCI	Spinal cord injured (patient)
SCMC	Sperm-cervical-mucus-contact (test)
SHBG	Sex hormone binding globulin
SPA	Sperm penetration assay
STD	Sexually transmitted disease
STI	Sexually transmitted infection
SUZI	Subzonal insemination
T3	Tri-iodothyronine
T4	Thyroxine
TAT	Tray agglutination test
TESA	Testicular sperm aspiration
TESE	Testicular sperm extraction
TEST	Tubal embryo stage transfer
TET	Tubal embryo transfer
TRH	Thyrotropin releasing hormone
TSH	Thyroid stimulating hormone
TUFT	Trans uterine fallopian transfer
UFO	Unfertilized oocyte
UTI	Urinary tract infection
VITI	Vaginal intratubal transfer
ZD	Zona drilling

Acronym	Meaning
ZIFT	Zygote intrafallopian transfer
ZPD	Zona pellucida drilling

Appendix I

Junaelo Institute of Reproductive Medicine
4256 Fulton Drive NW Suite B, Canton, Ohio 44718, USA
Tel: +1 (330) 497 9400
info@JunaeloReproductiveMedicine.com
www.JunaeloReproductiveMedicine.com

Medical History Form

Name: (First) _____ (Middle) _____ (Last) _____

Age: _____ Date of Birth: (Day/Month/Year) _____/ _____/ _____ Occupation: _____

Address: _____

City: _____ State/ZIP _____ Country _____

Home Tel: _____ Work Tel: _____ Mobile Tel: _____

E-mail: _____

Name of spouse/partner: _____

Age: _____ Date of Birth: (Day/Month/Year) _____/ _____/ _____ Occupation: _____

How long have you been trying to get pregnant?	
Is there any problem with sexual intercourse?	(Yes) (No) Details:
Has any cause been found for the infertility?	(Yes) (No) Details:
Which infertility investigations have you had and what were their results?	
Semen analysis ('sperm count') result	Count: _____ Motility: _____ Morphology: _____ Other comments:
Previous treatment for infertility and outcome	
Are your menstrual periods regular or irregular?	( ) Regular: Every 24-35 days ( ) Irregular cycles
Do you have any problems with your periods?	(Yes) (No) Details:

Are you allergic to any medication?   (Yes) (No) Details: _____

What medications are you taking right now?
_____

Personal Past/Present History
Have you had or do you currently suffer from any of the following diseases or any other disease/disorder that is not in the following list? Asthma, Ulcers, Pneumonia, Depression/anxiety, Chronic lung disease, Anemia/blood transfusion, Kidney infections/stones, Seizures/convulsions/epilepsy, Tuberculosis, Bowel trouble, Gonorrhea, Chlamydia, Herpes, Syphilis, Hepatitis B, Hepatitis C, Pelvic Inflammatory Disease, HIV/AIDS, Genital Warts, Arthritis/joint pain, Fracture, Jaundice, Diabetes, Thyroid gland problems, High blood pressure, Blood clot in leg/lungs, Stroke, Heart trouble/murmur, Rheumatic fever, Cancer, Breast lumps, Seizures, Mitral Valve Prolapse. If so provide details:

List any previous surgeries: _____

Previous hospitalizations: _____

OBSTETRIC HISTORY	Number		Number
Pregnancies		Miscarriages/Abortion	
Births		Ectopic/Tubal pregnancy	
Living children		Any pregnancy problems?	

SOCIAL HISTORY

	Yes	No			Would you like to quit?
Smoking	[]	[]	Packs per day ____	Years ____	[Yes] [No] [N/A]
Alcohol	[]	[]	Drinks per day ____	Per week ____	[Yes] [No] [N/A]
Drug use	[]	[]	Name ____	Years ____	[Yes] [No] [N/A]
Marital status	[] Married	[] Single	[] Widowed	[] Divorced	
School completed	[] Primary	[] Secondary	[] College/University	[] Other	

WOMAN'S PHYSICAL CHARACTERISTICS

Height: ____ meters; Weight: ____ Kg; Blood Pressure: ____ mm/Hg; Pulse: ____ /min

HUSBAND/SPOUSE

Have you had or do you currently suffer from any of the diseases that are outlined above or not included in the list: (Yes) (No) Explain: _____

Do you smoke? (Yes) (No). Do you drink alcohol? (Yes) (No). Do you use narcotic drugs? (Yes) (No).

DECLARATION

We hereby declare that the information supplied in this document accurately describes our medical history.

Woman's signature: .... **Man's signature:** ....**Date:** ....

Appendix II

Hysterosalpingography (HSG)

What is HSG?

HSG or hysterosalpingogram is a special X-ray photograph showing the out-line of the uterine cavity (inside of the womb) and the two fallopian tubes. The procedure (hysterosalpingography a.k.a. HSG) is used to determine whether a woman's tubes are open. It will also show whether there is anything that is distorting the shape of the uterine cavity such as uterine fibroids. HSG is one of the tests that are commonly carried out on infertile women to iden-tify the cause of the infertility.

At which part of the menstrual cycle is HSG performed?

The test is normally performed when the woman is most likely not pregnant. This is usually within the first 10 days of the menstrual cycle. The day on which the menstrual period starts is regarded as the first day (Day 1) of the cycle. The menstrual bleeding may last for 3-7 days in most women. HSG is not carried out while the bleeding is still present. It should be performed any-time from two days after the bleeding stops.

How to schedule the test

The physician normally requests HSG after the infertile couple consult him. The test is then scheduled at the hospital radiology department. The radiology department staff will give a definitive booking if the woman happens to be having her period at that time or had it recently and is still within the 10-day limit.

If already past Day 10 of the cycle, a tentative appointment is made for the next menstrual cycle based on the expected date of the next menstrual period. However, the woman has to inform the radiology department immediately her menstrual period starts to confirm the appointment.

How is HSG performed?

A gown is provided by the hospital for the patient to wear during the test. This is to avoid soiling or rumpling of her clothes. She lies down on a special table in the X-ray room and an instrument called a speculum is gently inserted into the vagina to allow the cervix (mouth of the womb) to be seen. The speculum is similar to the one that is used when a cervical smear (Pap smear) is performed.

The cervix is wiped clean of secretions and a pair of forceps clipped unto it. Slight traction is exerted on the cervix with the pair of forceps to straighten the angle between the cervix and the uterus. A cannula is then attached to the cervix; this is a tube through which the X-ray contrast dye is injected into the uterus. There are different types of cannulas but they serve the same function. Certain cannulas do not require the application of forceps on the cervix.

When the radiologist is ready, the patient's physician will slowly inject the special X-ray dye using the cannula. The radiologist will take pictures as the dye flows into the uterine cavity and hopefully through the fallopian tubes. If the tubes are open the dye will be seen to spill out of the fallopian tubes and into the pelvis.

Is HSG painful?

Different women have described their experience of HSG in different ways. Some say that it is 'just a little bit uncomfortable' whilst others say that it is painful. It appears that the major sensation felt by women during the test is that of uterine cramps. This is similar to the cramps that occur during the menstrual period. The most important thing to bear in mind is that the uncomfortable part of the test does not last long (about 30 seconds to one minute); every effort is made to reduce the discomfort.

How to prepare for the test

It is advisable to take a strong analgesic such as ibuprofen (600 mg all at once) or any other non-steroidal anti-inflammatory drug before HSG. The medication is taken about 1-2 hours before the test. This should decrease any discomfort felt during the test. Some patients can also be prescribed antibiotics to prevent pelvic infection. Apart from these, no other preparations are needed. The patient should report to the radiology department about 15 minutes before the test.

After the test

The patient rests for a short while before going home. She is advised to come with someone who will drive her home. She should not go back to work on that same day. The results of the test will be discussed at the next office visit.

Contraindications to HSG

The patient should not be pregnant at the time of the test. If there is a previous history of pelvic infection, another 'tubal patency test' such as laparoscopy and dye test should be performed instead. A history of allergy to iodine makes HSG unsafe because the X-ray dye that is used contains iodine. HSG should not be performed if the patient has vaginal bleeding.

Side effects and complications

Problems are rarely associated with HSG. However, there is a chance of pelvic infection. There may be an allergic reaction to the iodine-containing X-ray dye.

Comments

Hysterosalpingography is a relatively affordable and convenient test. It identifies a large proportion of women with tubal blockage. However, laparoscopy and dye test is often required to confirm findings made with HSG. Hysterosalpingography will not reveal any problems outside the fallopian tubes in the pelvis that may cause infertility such as endometriosis or scar tissue formation (adhesions). For this reason it is preferable to perform laparoscopy and dye test instead of HSG whenever possible. However, laparoscopy is a more expensive and inconvenient test than HSG.

Appendix III

Hysterosalpingocontrast sonography (HyCoSy)

This is a new type of test that is somewhat similar to hysterosalpingography (HSG). However, it does not involve the use of X-rays. Instead, the ultrasound scanner is used to monitor the flow of a special fluid that is slowly injected into the uterine cavity through the cervical canal. Ultrasound scanning is performed using a probe that is placed in the vagina. If the fallopian tubes are not blocked the fluid should be seen flowing through them.

Hysterosalpingocontrast sonography (HyCoSy) is still being evaluated but is not likely to be more accurate that the HSG. It is technically more difficult to perform and interpret compared to HSG. HyCoSy also suffers from a drawback similar to that of HSG in that the pelvis cannot be visualized. Therefore, HyCoSy cannot exclude the presence of adhesions in the pelvis even if the tubes are shown to be open. This is in contrast to laparoscopy and dye test.

Appendix IV

Laparoscopy and Dye (Chromotubation) Test

Aim

This procedure serves the purpose of checking for the patency of the fallopian tubes. It also provides an opportunity for the pelvis to be examined carefully, for the diagnosis of endometriosis, adhesions and any other problems that may cause or contribute to the state of infertility. Moreover, if performed in the luteal phase (second half) of the menstrual cycle evidence of ovulation in that cycle may be found; this helps to confirm that the woman is ovulating normally.

Caution

Care should be taken to ensure that the woman is not pregnant if the test is to be carried out in the luteal phase of the menstrual cycle. The couple is asked to use barrier contraceptives such as condoms during the fertile period of that cycle. It is also prudent to perform a sensitive pregnancy test on the day of the procedure

A day-case procedure

Laparoscopy and dye test is usually performed as a day-case procedure. The patient comes to the hospital on the morning of the procedure fasting from midnight. Her partner, an adult relative or a friend should accompany her. This precaution is important because she will need someone to drive her home or accompany her if she has to use the public transport system, after the operation.

Anesthesia

Laparoscopy is normally carried out under general anesthesia. The administered drugs are short lasting and full consciousness is regained soon after the procedure. Laparoscopy can also be performed under local anesthesia or "conscious sedation".

Procedure

After establishing adequate anesthesia, a special needle is inserted into the abdominal cavity through a small incision (<1 cm) that is made just below the umbilicus. Two to three liters of carbon dioxide gas are introduced through this needle to distend the abdomen and make it easier to see the pelvic organs

A laparoscope is a rigid metal viewing tube that is connected to a video camera and TV monitor. It is inserted into the abdominal cavity through this incision and used in inspecting the ovaries, tubes and uterus. The pelvis itself is also inspected carefully, looking for evidence of endometriosis and adhesions. Another incision is made lower down the abdomen; this is for the introduction of instruments that are used in maneuvering the pelvic organs to permit their complete examination.

The dye test (a.k.a. chromotubation) is carried out with the laparoscope still positioned in the abdomen. A cannula is connected to the cervical canal and methylene blue dye slowly injected. The blue dye is seen to distend the tubes and then flow out of the open end of the fallopian tubes if the tubes are not blocked.

Afterwards, the carbon dioxide gas is removed from the abdomen and the small incision(s) closed with one or two absorbable stitches. The patient is allowed home accompanied, after resting for some hours. She may feel slightly bloated and uncomfortable but this settles within a day or two. She should rest at home for a few days (two to three days) before resuming work.

Complications

Laparoscopy is relatively safe but complications are possible. Any of the abdominal or pelvic organs, including bowel and blood vessels, can be damaged during insertion of the instruments. If the damage is substantial, a formal operating procedure may be required for the repair of the traumatized organ and the patient will need to stay in hospital longer than initially anticipated.

Some of the carbon dioxide may enter the blood stream as gas bubbles and reach the heart and lungs before being completely dissolved in the blood. This is called embolism and it is a desperate emergency condition. Embolism is not common with carbon dioxide; it is more common when other gases such as room air or nitrogen are used in place of carbon dioxide for laparoscopy.

Not all the carbon dioxide gas can be removed from the abdominal cavity after laparoscopy; the remaining gas will be slowly absorbed by the body and this may take more than one day for this to be completed. During that time some of the gas will remain under the patient's diaphragm and irritate it especially when she is sitting up or standing.

Because of the origin of the nerve supply to the diaphragm the irritation will be felt as shoulder tip pain. The pain is however, self-limiting and will disappear after some time.

Another complication is that of carrying out laparoscopy and dye test in the presence of an early pregnancy. This is an uncommon complication and there is not much information on what happens to that pregnancy but it seems that it usually continues without problems. The couple must use barrier contraceptives for sexual intercourse in the month the woman has this procedure or abstain from sex. Furthermore, a pregnancy test should be performed in all cases just prior to laparoscopy.

Laparoscopy and dye test compared with other tubal patency tests

Hysterosalpingogram (HSG) and hysterosalpingocontrast sonography (HyCoSy) are two other tests of tubal patency. They are less expensive to carry out compared to laparoscopy and dye test; the patient remains awake during the tests. No incisions are required and there are fewer complications.

However, HSG and HyCoSy: (1) will not identify all cases of tubal blockage; (2) results can at times be difficult to interpret; (3) may lead to a diagnosis of tubal blockage where none exists (false positive result); and, (4) do not provide any information on whether there are adhesions, endometriosis or any other pelvic lesions that affect fertility.

It is therefore impossible to exclude such causes of infertility in a patient who has not had laparoscopy even though the HSG (or HyCoSy) was normal. Laparoscopy and dye test is often required to clarify abnormal results obtained with the other two investigations. Whenever possible laparoscopy and dye test should be performed instead of HSG and HyCoSy.

Appendix V

Instructions to Patients for Producing Semen Samples by Masturbation

- You need to abstain from sexual intercourse and ejaculation for 2-3 days. The period of abstinence must not exceed five days since longer periods will not improve the sperm count. Rather there will be more dead sperm in the ejaculate.

- You can produce the semen sample at home but it is preferable to produce it in the laboratory where a special room has been reserved. Magazines and videos are kept in this room for those who wish to use them.

- If you produce the sample at home make sure the container is not placed in a hot or cold place since temperature extremes will kill the sperm. Bring the semen sample to the laboratory as soon as possible after producing the sample; the sample should reach the laboratory within one hour of production.

- Produce the sample by masturbation. Prior to this, wash your hands and genitals with soap and rinse thoroughly with water then dry with a clean towel. Please do not use any lubricant for masturbation, as most lubricants are toxic to sperm.

- Ejaculate directly into the plastic container that has been given to you. If you have any problems with scheduling the test or producing the semen sample please tell your physician.

Appendix VI

Steps in the Treatment with Intrauterine Insemination (IUI)

1. You will be given drugs to stimulate your ovaries to produce 2-4 eggs.

2. The first drug is clomiphene citrate tablet. Each tablet contains 50 mg. You will take one or two tablets (as directed by the Physician) every morning on Days 2, 3, 4, 5 and 6 of your menstrual cycle (i.e. for five days). You will not take clomiphene citrate tablets after this time.

3. Some patients may be administered gonadotropin injections in addition; they have various brand names. The dose is 1-2 ampules of the injection on Days 5 and 7.

4. You will then have an ultrasound scan on Day 9. After reviewing the results of the scan the physician may ask you to have gonadotropin injection on that same day and on specific days afterwards.

5. You will have ultrasound scans at different intervals during the treatment. Most of the ultrasound scans are performed through the vagina.

6. In order to determine when ovulation will take place, a test will be carried out using your urine sample. You will be told when to start this test. Usually it will be performed everyday from about Day 9. If the test result becomes positive, it means that you will ovulate within 40 hours (sometimes 24 hours). Phone your physician immediately so that he can arrange for you to come for the insemination.

7. If however, the test is still negative but the ultrasound scan shows that your eggs are ready to be released we will give you an injection of human chorionic gonadotropin (HCG) (various brand names). This will make your ovaries release the eggs about 36 hours later. HCG injection can also be given to you when you notice the urine test become positive. This will ensure that your ovaries release all the eggs.

8. When the eggs are ready to be ovulated you will come to the Institute for insemination.

9. Your partner will produce a semen sample about two hours before the insemination. This will be processed in the laboratory so that only normal motile sperm are used.

10. The prepared sperm will be placed inside your uterus using a thin plastic tube that is attached to a syringe. To do this some instruments (e.g. vaginal speculum) will have to be placed in your vagina for a few minutes just like is done when you have a vaginal examination for Pap smear.

11. You will lie on the couch for a few minutes afterwards to allow the sperm spread out in your uterus and begin to move towards the fallopian tubes where they hopefully should meet the eggs.

12. The insemination will be carried out either once or on two consecutive days, depending on patient characteristics and other aspects of the treatment cycle.

13. Afterwards continue with life as usual. There are no special instructions. Come to the Institute two weeks after the insemination for a pregnancy test. This will be performed on a urine sample or a sample of blood that is withdrawn from you. The results may be available within a few minutes, so you can wait for the result. If the test takes longer to perform the Physician or nurse will phone you on that same day with the test results. Please note that your periods may start a few days before this test if you are not pregnant. In that case, call and cancel the pregnancy test.

    Wishing you the best of luck!

Appendix VII

Treatment Schedule and Instructions for Intrauterine Insemination using Clomiphene Citrate

DAY OF MENSTRUAL CYCLE	DAY/DATE	COMMENTS/INSTRUCTION
1		Your menses started today. Phone the Institute.
2		• Take _____ mg Clomiphene citrate tablet(s)
3		• Take _____ mg Clomiphene citrate tablet(s)
4		• Take _____ mg Clomiphene citrate tablet(s)
5		• Take _____ mg Clomiphene citrate tablet(s)
6		• Take _____ mg Clomiphene citrate tablet(s)
7		No medication today
8		No medication today

DAY OF MENSTRUAL CYCLE	DAY/DATE	COMMENTS/INSTRUCTION
9		• Testing of urine for ovulation prediction (phone the Institute if positive) • ULTRASOUND SCAN
10		• Testing of urine for ovulation prediction (phone the Institute if positive)
11		• Testing of urine for ovulation prediction (phone the Institute if positive) • ULTRASOUND SCAN
12		• Testing of urine for ovulation prediction (phone the Institute if positive) • ?ULTRASOUND SCAN
13		• Testing of urine for ovulation prediction (phone the Institute if positive) • ULTRASOUND SCAN
?		? Human chorionic gonadotropin injection
?		? Insemination #1
?		? Insemination #2
Two weeks after IUI		Come for a test to find out if you are pregnant. If your menses start before this date it is most likely that you are not pregnant.

<u>NOTE</u>

If the ovulation prediction test becomes positive, it means that you shall ovulate within the next 36-40 hours. You should phone the Institute immediately you get that result to arrange a time for you to come with your partner to the Institute for IUI. If we can, we will give you an injection of HCG immediately the prediction test becomes positive.

If the ovulation prediction urine test does not become positive, HCG injection will be given to make you ovulate when the ultrasound scan demonstrates that you are ready for the injection. It is important that you have the HCG injection at the exact time.

The dose of clomiphene citrate and the sequence of ultrasound scans may change during the treatment cycle.

Appendix VIII

Treatment Schedule and Instructions for Intrauterine Insemination using Clomiphene Citrate and Gonadotropins

DAY OF MENSTRUAL CYCLE	DAY/DATE	COMMENTS/INSTRUCTION
1		Your menses started today. Phone the Institute.
2		• Take _____ mg Clomiphene citrate tablet(s)
3		• Take _____ mg Clomiphene citrate tablet(s)
4		• Take _____ mg Clomiphene citrate tablet(s)
5		• Take _____ mg Clomiphene citrate tablet(s) • _____ ampule(s) of gonadotropin injection
6		• Take _____ mg Clomiphene citrate tablet(s)
7		• _____ ampule(s) of gonadotropin injection

DAY OF MENSTRUAL CYCLE	DAY/DATE	COMMENTS/INSTRUCTION
8		No tablet or injection today
9		• Testing of urine for ovulation prediction (phone the Institute if positive) • ULTRASOUND SCAN • _____ ampule(s) of gonadotropin injection after scan
10		• Testing of urine for ovulation prediction (phone the Institute if positive)
11		• Testing of urine for ovulation prediction (phone the Institute if positive) • ULTRASOUND SCAN • _____ ampule(s) of gonadotropin injection
12		• Testing of urine for ovulation prediction (phone the Institute if positive) • ULTRASOUND SCAN • _____ ampule(s) of gonadotropin injection
13		• Testing of urine for ovulation prediction (phone the Institute if positive) • ULTRASOUND SCAN • _____ ampule(s) of gonadotropin injection
?		? Human chorionic gonadotropin injection
?		? Insemination #1
?		? Insemination #2
Two weeks after insemination		Come for a test to find out if you are pregnant. We will call you with the results. If your menses start before this date it is most likely that you are not pregnant.

<u>NOTE</u>

If the ovulation prediction test becomes positive, it means that you shall ovulate within the next 36 hours. You should phone the Institute immediately you get that result to arrange a time for you to come with your partner to the Institute for IUI. If we can, we will give you an injection of HCG immediately the prediction test becomes positive.

If the ovulation prediction urine test does not become positive, HCG injection will be given to make you ovulate when the ultrasound scan demonstrates that you are ready for the injection. It is important that you have the HCG injection at the exact time.

The dose and sequence of tablets and injections may be changed by the physician based on the ultrasound scan results and other factors.

Appendix IX

General instructions for drug administration

- Day 1 of the menstrual cycle is the first day of proper blood flow. Any pre-menstrual spotting is to be ignored. If the menstrual loss starts late in the evening, consider the next day as Day 1 and follow the protocol accordingly.

- We prefer to do ultrasound scans using the internal (vaginal) technique as this gives a clearer and more accurate assessment. For this internal scan, the bladder has to be empty. In some cases, an abdominal scan will be indicated and you will be advised to have a full bladder.

- If you have been prescribed Synarel (Nafarelin) nasal spray, ensure that it is applied regularly at the exact times indicated.

- Ensure that the gonadotropin hormone injections are given at approximately the same time each day (within a period of two hours).

- Please remember to bring your drug administration sheet with you every time you come for an injection.

- "One ampule" = one ampule of the drug (e.g. Follistim, Gonal-F or Repronex). Up to six ampules of the drug can be dissolved in 1 ml of the solvent.

- These drugs do not necessarily need to be kept in the fridge; a cool cupboard or drawer will suffice. However long term storage instructions may vary depending on the specific medication. Please read the drug inserts for more information.

- We can administer your injections during our working hours. You will be given the exact time to come for your injections.

- Please try to avoid the lunch-time period if at all possible (i.e. 12:00–13:00 hours) as this can be a very busy time.

- However, on days when you would not otherwise be required to attend the Institute, you may find it more convenient if arrangements can be made through your own family physician for the administration of these injections.

- We usually teach most of our patients and their spouses how to administer the drugs by themselves. This method appears to be the best as it is much more convenient for you.

- Should you have an ultrasound scan and an injection on the same day, please ensure that you have your scan first as the drug dosage may change. It is worth bringing extra drugs with you on ultrasound scan days even if you are not due to have an injection, since the drug schedule may be changed depending on your response to the drugs.

- The dose of your drug may be written as 'IU' (i.e. international units) instead of as 'ampules'.

- If you have any concerns about the treatment, please do not hesitate to contact your physician or nurse at the Institute for advice.

Appendix X

In Vitro Fertilization Treatment Schedule and Instructions

TREATMENT CYCLE DAY	DAY/DATE	COMMENTS/INSTRUCTION
0 minus		You may be given oral contraceptive or other tablets to readjust your menstrual cycle. This may not be necessary for every patient.
0 minus		GnRHa (e.g. Lupron, Lupron Depot, Zoladex or Nafarelin) administration starts.
0 minus		Baseline ultrasound scan (Time = ...). Blood tests. Final instructions and consents.
?		Pre-anesthetic clinic review by the anesthetist.
1		_____ IU of gonadotropin injection.
2		_____ IU of gonadotropin injection.
3		_____ IU of gonadotropin injection.
4		_____ IU of gonadotropin injection.

TREATMENT CYCLE DAY	DAY/DATE	COMMENTS/INSTRUCTION
5		_____ IU of gonadotropin injection.
6		Ultrasound scan (Time = ...). Blood test. _____ IU of gonadotropin injection .
7		_____ IU of gonadotropin injection.
8		Ultrasound scan (Time = ...). _____ IU of gonadotropin injection.
9		_____ IU of gonadotropin injection.
10		Ultrasound scan (Time = ...). _____ IU of gonadotropin injection.
11		?? Ultrasound scan (Time = ...). ?? _____ IU of gonadotropin injection. ?? _____ IU of HCG injection.
12		?
13		?
14		?
15		?
?		10,000 IU of HCG injection. You **must** have this injection **exactly** by .... p.m.
? + 1		Rest day. No food or fluid after midnight.

TREATMENT CYCLE DAY	DAY/DATE	COMMENTS/INSTRUCTION
? + 2		Report to the Institute. Egg collection will be done this morning by ......a.m. Husband to provide semen sample this morning. Go home later today. Start inserting progesterone suppositories **tonight**.
? + 3		Institute staff will phone you today with the fertilization result. You may be given a time to come in tomorrow for the embryo transfer. Remember to insert progesterone suppositories twice a day.
? + 4		Insert progesterone suppositories into the rectum this morning. Embryo transfer may take place today. Time ....
		Continue inserting progesterone suppositories twice a day.
Two weeks after IVF		Come for a blood test to find out if you are pregnant. If your menses start before this date it is most likely that you are not pregnant. Call us.

Wishing you the best of luck in your treatment.

Appendix XI

After the egg retrieval

- Now that your egg recovery is over, the next most important step is for us to establish whether fertilization has occurred. Our Laboratory will be monitoring your eggs during the next 24 hours to see whether there are positive signs that fertilization has taken place.

- One of us will telephone you tomorrow to tell you whether fertilization has occurred. We will also tell you when to come for embryo transfer.

- When you attend the Institute on the day of embryo transfer, we will review the treatment progress and confirm that your embryos have started dividing and can be transferred into your womb on that same day.

- We sometimes need to use ultrasound directed embryo replacement techniques to make the transfer easier so we ask you not to empty your bladder once you have arrived at the Institute.

- You may notice a slight vaginal blood loss or blood stained urine. This will usually clear itself quite quickly but if you have any anxiety whatsoever, then please do not hesitate to call your physician or nurse at the Institute.

- You may also notice that your abdomen may look quite swollen. This is also normal and should resolve within a few days, but if you are worried, please call us.

- We wish you every success in your attempt at achieving a pregnancy.

Appendix XII

Progesterone administration following egg collection

- We recommend that patients receive progesterone supplementation starting in the evening of this same day in which egg collection was carried out. This is to ensure that their progesterone level remains at a high value thereby assisting with implantation.

- Insert the progesterone suppositories into the vagina twice a day at regular intervals (i.e. morning and evening), starting with the first one this evening.

- Continue until you return for your pregnancy blood test. If you are pregnant, the suppositories should be continued until three months of pregnancy.

- On the day of your embryo transfer, please insert the suppository rectally. After the embryo transfer please resume inserting the suppositories into the vagina.

- In a small percentage of patients undergoing IVF, fertilization will not occur. In these circumstances, it will not be necessary to continue with the progesterone suppositories.

- We wish you every success in your attempt at achieving a pregnancy.

Appendix XIII

After the embryo transfer

- Now that the embryo transfer has been undertaken, we wish you every success with this attempt.

- You will have been prescribed a course of progesterone suppositories that are given to you to try to maximize the prospects of success. There is a suggestion that progesterone supplementation will assist implantation of the embryo.

- After the embryo transfer, we suggest you conduct your daily life in a routine manner. There is no evidence to suggest that any specific activity will influence the outcome of in vitro fertilization treatment. This includes having sexual intercourse. However, you may elect to refrain from having sex until you feel completely comfortable after the egg recovery procedure.

- If you have any embryos remaining after the embryo transfer, the Laboratory will assess them. If they are found suitable for freezing this will be carried out. We normally should be able to tell you immediately if there are embryos for freezing.

- The next important step is to establish whether pregnancy has occurred. This can be determined by having a urine or blood test on the 14th day following the egg retrieval.

- There is a possibility that the course of medications you are on such as progesterone may delay the onset of your menstrual period for a few days.

- We can also arrange for an early ultrasound scan to be carried out to confirm the pregnancy when the menstrual period is two weeks overdue. If you live some distance away, you may wish to have this done locally.

- We ask if you would kindly get in touch with the Institute when you know the outcome of this attempt, whether successful or otherwise. Call us at the Institute by telephone.

- We would like you to have a consultation at our clinic irrespective of the outcome.

Appendix XIV

Outcome of treatment form

- We wish you every success with your treatment. We would be very grateful if you would kindly complete and return the section below when you discover whether you have become pregnant.

- We would appreciate it if you could return this form even if you have already telephoned to let us know whether you are pregnant or not. The reason for this is to obtain accurate results of all treatment cycles undertaken, whether successful or unsuccessful, so these can be monitored and this, we hope, will assist us in striving to achieve further successes.

- If pregnancy does occur, we can make arrangements for your immediate supportive care.

- We will arrange an ultrasound scan two weeks after the positive test. This is to establish whether the pregnancy is viable and if so, the number of embryos that have been implanted.

- If the pregnancy is on-going, we will advise continuation of the progesterone medication.

- If pregnancy unfortunately does not occur on this occasion, we appreciate the anxiety this might cause. We would be pleased to see you for a follow-up consultation. This is to discuss your most recent treatment and plan for future management. You are welcome to contact the nurses or physician in either situation.

- Thank you for your cooperation.

NAME:

_____

REGISTRATION NO.

_____

ADDRESS:

_____

_____

TELEPHONE NO:

DATE OF

_____

PROCEDURE:

IUI/IVF/ICSI/GIFT/FER/

_____

ZIFT/OTHER (_please_

state)

IF PREGNANT

_____

Date confirmed

_____

Number of fetuses

_____

ANY COMMENTS

_____

_____

Appendix XV

Why we recommend an ultrasound scan 2-3 weeks after your positive pregnancy test (6-7 weeks pregnant)

To confirm viability

Although positive βHCG pregnancy test results show that implantation has occurred, the multiplication of the embryonic cells may infrequently cease at any time in early pregnancy. This could result in the presence of a pregnancy sac within the uterus but no fetal pole. This is referred to as a blighted ovum.

To confirm viability, a gestation sac (black circle on ultrasound scan), a fetal pole (bright shadow within the black sac) and a fetal heart beat (a pulsation within the bright shadow) must be identified.

To determine the number of fetuses

Although most positive tests are due to a singleton pregnancy, twins or triplets may occur. An ultrasound scan can identify the number of gestation sacs and fetuses present.

CAN THE SCAN BE PERFORMED EARLIER?

An earlier scan can still identify the pregnancy sac(s) but the embryo is too small to be positively identified. Since a further scan is needed to confirm the presence of a fetal pole, and hence the viability of the pregnancy, we recommend the scan be performed not earlier than three weeks after the positive pregnancy result (seven weeks pregnant).

Further scans are recommended at eight weeks after the pregnancy test (12 weeks pregnant), and at 19 and 32 weeks of pregnancy.

The full duration of a pregnancy up to term is 40 weeks, starting from the first day of the last menstrual period (LMP) in a natural cycle. Hence, in a controlled cycle, the LMP date is two weeks prior to the procedure date.

Appendix XVI

Outcome of pregnancy report form

Patient's name:	
Patient's date of birth:	
Treatment date:	
Did your pregnancy result in the birth of live baby/babies?	
If so, on what day was/were your baby/babies born?	
How much did he/she/they weigh?	
What is the sex of your baby/babies?	
Did your labor start normally, or did your doctor induce you?	
Did you have a cesarean section?	
Was/were your baby/babies born with any abnormality? (*Please specify*)	
Did your pregnancy unfortunately end in miscarriage, or any other complication? If so, please give details.	
Thank you for your cooperation. Please mail the completed form to the Institute	

Appendix XVII

Frozen Embryo Replacement: Treatment Schedule and Instructions

TREATMENT CYCLE DAY	DAY/DATE	COMMENTS/INSTRUCTIONS
0 minus		• You may be given tablets to readjust your menstrual cycle. This will not be necessary for every patient.
0 minus		• GnRHa (e.g. Lupron, Lupron Depot, Zoladex, Nafarelin) administration starts.
0 minus		• Baseline ultrasound scan (Time = ...) • Blood tests, final instructions and consents.
1		• 2 mg tablet of Estradiol taken twice a day.
2		• 2 mg tablet of Estradiol taken twice a day.
3		• 2 mg tablet of Estradiol taken twice a day.
4		• 2 mg tablet of Estradiol taken twice a day.
5		• 2 mg tablet of Estradiol taken twice a day.
6		• 2 mg tablet of Estradiol taken twice a day.
7		• 2 mg tablet of Estradiol taken twice a day.
8		• 2 mg tablet of Estradiol taken THREE TIMES a day.
9		• 2 mg tablet of Estradiol taken THREE TIMES a day.
10		• 2 mg tablet of Estradiol taken THREE TIMES a day.
11		• 2 mg tablet of Estradiol taken THREE TIMES a day.

TREATMENT CYCLE DAY	DAY/DATE	COMMENTS/INSTRUCTIONS
12		• 2 mg tablet of Estradiol taken THREE TIMES a day.
13		• 2 mg tablet of Estradiol taken THREE TIMES a day.
14		• 2 mg tablet of Estradiol taken THREE TIMES a day. • Stop using GnRHa. • Ultrasound scan (Time = ...).
15		• 2 mg tablet of Estradiol taken THREE TIMES a day. • 200 mg progesterone suppository inserted twice a day.
16		• 2 mg tablet of Estradiol taken THREE TIMES a day. • 200 mg progesterone suppository inserted twice a day.
17		• 2 mg tablet of Estradiol taken THREE TIMES a day. • 200 mg progesterone suppository inserted twice a day. • <u>Insert progesterone suppository into the rectum this morning.</u> • Embryo transfer should normally take place today. • Time ....
From Day 18 until pregnancy test		• 2 mg tablet of Estradiol taken THREE TIMES a day. • 200 mg progesterone suppository inserted twice a day.
Two weeks after embryo transfer		• Come for a blood test to find out if you are pregnant. • If your menses start before this date it is most likely that you are not pregnant. Call us. If after talking with you we are sure you are having your menses we will instruct you to stop using Estradiol and Progesterone. • If the pregnancy test result shows that you are pregnant, you will need to continue with Estradiol tablets (2 mg tablet of Estradiol taken THREE TIMES a day) and Progesterone suppositories (200 mg twice daily) until you are 12 weeks pregnant

Wishing you the best of luck in your treatment.

Appendix XVIII

Finally!

Please inform your physician and nurse of the pregnancy outcome. It is important for couples to keep in touch with the fertility unit and notify them of the outcome of their pregnancy. This will help in keeping accurate records, which have formed the basis for most research that is carried out in this area. Such research aims at improving further the results of treatment. In some countries, it is required by law that fertility centers should notify the regulatory agency of the outcome of treatment of their patients.

The medical team knows all their patients by name and remain interested in their welfare long after they have completed their treatment and become pregnant. Although it is not happy news they would still like to know if their patients miscarry, have ectopic pregnancies or any other undesirable outcome. They are happy when they hear that one of their patients delivered recently. They are even happier when pictures of the babies start arriving and they eventually visit the unit with their parents.

It is not just the babies; pictures of toddlers, young children, adolescents and recently, adults, adorn the walls of many units. These act as testimony of the work that is being carried out at infertility treatment facilities to help infertile couples obtain one of life's greatest gifts.

Appendix XIX

Junaelo Institute of Reproductive Medicine
4256 Fulton Drive NW Suite B, Canton, Ohio 44718, USA
Tel: +1 (330) 497 9400
info@JunaeloReproductiveMedicine.com
www.JunaeloReproductiveMedicine.com

Donor Lifestyle Declaration
(Adapted from a public domain document)

An Important Notice to All Donors

There are some people in the community who must not donate gametes (sperm and eggs) because their lifestyle may give rise to conditions that would be detrimental to children born of their sperm/eggs or result in infections in the patients who receive them. If in doubt, please consult the staff at the Institute.

In the light of the present knowledge of AIDS (Acquired Immune Deficiency Syndrome) and although a screening test is currently performed on all gamete donors, people in the at-risk groups must not to donate. These people are:

- Intravenous drug users (at any time in the past five years).
- Prostitutes of either sex (and their clients).
- Sexual partners of the above or of bisexual males.

Statement by Person Intending to Donate Sperm or Eggs

I, ... (Name of Donor)
of, ... (Address of Donor)
do hereby declare that, to the best of my knowledge:

1. I am not carrying the viruses or suffering from AIDS (Acquired Immune Deficiency Syndrome) or any disease related to it;
2. I am not suffering from night sweats, unintentional weight loss, persistent fever, diarrhea or swollen glands;
3. I have not engaged in male to male sexual activity during the last five years.
4. I have not injected myself, or been injected with, any drug not prescribed for me by a registered medical or dental practitioner within the past five years;
5. I have not received a blood transfusion or treatment with human blood products within the past five years.

6. Neither my spouse nor any sexual partner comes within the categories described in items 1,2,3,4 and 5.
7. I have no communicable disease and I have never suffered from such an ailment in the past, except as follows: ....
8. I am in good health and I have never suffered from any physical, mental or psychological impediment, disability or abnormality whether inherited or as a result of any disease, ailment or accident, except as follows:
   ....
9. I am aware of the possible transmission of inheritable diseases and neither I nor any of my relatives have had any such conditions (except those indicated):
   ....
10. I have not been tattooed within the past five years.
11. I have not had jaundice or hepatitis in the past twelve months or been in close contact with any person suffering from those diseases within the past six months.
12. I am signing this statement in the presence of a member of the staff of the Institute.

Name of Donor: .... Signature: ....

Name of Witness: .... Signature: ....

If an individual is unable to give a clear declaration in response to all of the above statements before sperm or eggs are donated, a physician must interview the donor. I, ... (Name of Physician) have interviewed .... and have found no reason why he/she should not donate sperm/eggs.

Signature of Physician: .... Date: ..../........./..................

Appendix XX

Junaelo Institute of Reproductive Medicine
4256 Fulton Drive NW Suite B, Canton, Ohio 44718, USA

Tel: +1 (330) 497 9400

info@JunaeloReproductiveMedicine.com

www.JunaeloReproductiveMedicine.com

Egg Donor Genetic Screening Form				
Familial conditions	Donor	Mother	Father	Siblings
Alcoholism				
Alzheimer's disease				
Blindness				
Deafness/Hearing loss				
Depression or mania				
Diabetes with onset at young age				
Epilepsy				
Heart disease				
Hypertension				
Schizophrenia				
Severe arthritis				
Any other condition (specify)				
Malformations				
Cleft lip or palate				
Clubfoot				
Heart defect				
Spina bifida				
Any other condition (specify)				
Mendelian disorders				
Color blindness				
Cystic fibrosis				
Glaucoma				
Hemophilia				
Huntington's disease				
Muscular dystrophy				
Polycystic kidneys				
Sickle cell anemia				
Tay-Sachs disease				
Any other condition (specify)				

Note: Adapted from Sauer MV, Cohen MA. Egg Donation. In *Textbook of Assisted Reproductive Techniques Laboratory and Clinical Perspectives.* (Gardner DK, Weissman A, Howles CM, Shoham Z. eds.). Martin Dunitz Ltd, London. pp.691-701.

Appendix XXI

Junaelo Institute of Reproductive Medicine
4256 Fulton Drive NW Suite B, Canton, Ohio 44718, USA

Tel: +1 (330) 497 9400

info@JunaeloReproductiveMedicine.com

www.JunaeloReproductiveMedicine.com

Egg Donor's Family Background

Relation	Age if living	Age at death	Cause of death
Grandfather (paternal)			
Grandmother (paternal)			
Grandfather (maternal)			
Grandmother (maternal)			
Father			
Mother			
Brothers			
Sisters			

Note: Adapted from Sauer MV, Cohen MA. Egg Donation. In *Textbook of Assisted Reproductive Techniques Laboratory and Clinical Perspectives*. (Gardner DK, Weissman A, Howles CM, Shoham Z. eds.). Martin Dunitz Ltd, London. pp.691-701.

Appendix XXII

Junaelo Institute of Reproductive Medicine
4256 Fulton Drive NW Suite B, Canton, Ohio 44718, USA

Tel: +1 (330) 497 9400

info@JunaeloReproductiveMedicine.com
www.JunaeloReproductiveMedicine.com

Egg Donor's Ethnic Background

Relation	Ethnicity/Race
Father	
Grandfather (paternal)	
Grandmother (paternal)	
Great grandfather (paternal)	
Great grandmother (paternal)	
Mother	
Grandfather (maternal)	
Grandmother (maternal)	
Great grandfather (maternal)	
Great grandmother (maternal)	

Index

Afterword

I have enjoyed writing this book. This is a work in evolution so I will welcome comments and other feedback that can be incorporated in future editions of the book. Send these by email to info@JunaeloReproductiveMedicine.com. You can also visit our website at http://www.JunaeloReproductiveMedicine.com for more information on this and other publications. This site also has a wealth of information on infertility and reproductive healthcare. I wish you success in all endeavors arising from the information you obtained from this book.

Godwin I. Meniru, M.D.

About the Author

Dr. Godwin I. Meniru obtained his medical degree, with Distinction in Pharmacology, from the University of Nigeria in 1984. He then underwent categorical residencies in Obstetrics and Gynecology in England, Nigeria and the USA. He also completed a full time course of studies at the University of Nottingham leading to the award of the Master of Medical Sciences degree in Assisted Reproduction Technology. He became a Member of the Royal College of Obstetricians and Gynaecologists in 1995. He is also a foundation Member of the Faculty of Family Planning and Reproductive Health Care of the Royal College of Obstetricians and Gynaecologists.

Dr. Meniru's subspecialty training included a Fellowship in Reproductive Medicine at the London Fertility Centre, Harley Street, from 1995 to 1997 under the supervision of Professor Ian Craft. In addition to being a clinician, he is a fully trained embryologist and andrologist and licensed to perform intracytoplasmic sperm injection by the Human Fertilisation and Embryology Authority of England.

Dr. Meniru worked as a Consultant in the Department of Reproductive Medicine of the Royal Brunei Jerudong Park Medical Centre, Brunei Darussalam, Southeast Asia from 1997 to 1999. He directed the andrology laboratory program as well as co-directing the clinical in vitro fertilization program. He achieved high treatment success rates for his infertility patients and was responsible for introducing surgical sperm retrieval as well as other innovations into the program.

Dr. Godwin Meniru now lives in the United States of America with his family. He founded the Junaelo Institute of Reproductive Medicine to provide a wide range of reproductive healthcare and infertility treatment. The Institute also provides advanced reproductive therapy including in vitro fertilization treatment. Dr. Meniru is an Assistant Professor of Obstetrics and Gynecology at the Northeastern Ohio Universities College of Medicine.

Dr. Meniru has researched extensively in Reproductive Medicine, Obstetrics and Gynecology. He has written or co-authored more than 120 scientific papers, abstracts and book chapters. He edited and was the principal author of *A Handbook of Intrauterine Insemination*, which was published by Cambridge University Press in 1997. He is the sole author of another book, *Cambridge Guide to Infertility Management and Assisted Reproduction* also published by the Cambridge University Press, in 2001. The Writers Advantage Press published his third book *Prevention of Infertility and Complications in Women: A Comprehensive Guide to the Preservation of Female Reproductive Health*. He has broad ranging research interests in Reproductive Medicine and preventive health care.

Contact Information

Junaelo Institute of Reproductive Medicine
4256 Fulton Drive NW Suite B, Canton, Ohio 44718, USA
Tel: +1 (330) 497 9400
E-mail address: info@JunaeloReproductiveMedicine.com
Web site: www.JunaeloReproductiveMedicine.com

0-595-33089-4

www.ingramcontent.com/pod-product-compliance
Lightning Source LLC
Chambersburg PA
CBHW031049180526
45163CB00002BA/758